MW00905082

Life
Isn't Meant to Be a
Struggle!

*A Journey of
Self-Discovery and
Transformation*

FRANCESCA TOMAS

ISBN - 13: 978-0-9964460-4-4
ISBN - 10: 0-9964460-4-4

This publication is designed to provide accurate and authoritative information in regard to the subject matter covered. It is sold with the understanding that the publisher is not engaged in rendering medical, legal, accounting, or other professional services.

If medical advice or other expert assistance is required, the services of a competent professional person should be sought.

Published by: Expert Author Publishing
http://expertauthorpublishing.com
Canadian Address:
Expert Author Publishing
1108 - 1155 The High Street,
Coquitlam, BC, Canada
V3B 7W4
Phone: (604) 941-3041
Fax: (604) 944-7993

US Address:
1300 Boblett Street
Unit A-218
Blaine, WA 98230
Phone: (866) 492-6623
Fax: (250) 493-6603

Printed in Surrey, British Columbia by CanEngrave Signs and Printing

Dedication

This book is possible because of the many clients who have come through my doors seeking help. They have willingly opened their minds and hearts to a new way of thinking about their life journeys. Your generosity of spirit has helped me grow both as a counsellor and as a person. Thank you.

I love the wonderful men in my life! I must give thanks to my husband and my two sons. I appreciate your understanding and support as we ride through life in tandem.

Table of Contents

Introduction

My gut told me to write this book. It's that simple. Over the years, I have learned to trust messages that come from this deep inner level. I understood that I was meant to share my blessings with a bigger audience. What you will read here are the lessons I have learned.

At the end of the book, I will explain how to get in touch with me if you would like to continue the adventure and take your learning to another level.

My passion for writing this book comes from my wish to share how to become really connected to your inner self. I want you to learn how to enjoy your own company and have the profound experience of truly loving yourself.

I will show you a simple system I've used successfully in my practice as a therapist to help many people transform their unhappy lives to happy ones.

The S.T.A.R. system is a product of my experience as a counsellor helping others, as a student learning from formal and informal sources, and most importantly, as a person. I underwent my own transformation. In my early twenties, I was a confused and uncertain young woman who couldn't work for a year because of my personal issues. I will explain that soon. With lots of hard work, I became an accomplished, confident, and independent woman. I now seek continual learning and growth in my life and see them as necessary.

Although I have been working as a counsellor with all of these concepts for years, the S.T.A.R. acronym came to me while I was on a plane. Did being closer to the stars while up there in the stratosphere influence my thinking? Anything is possible!

This book addresses some difficult topics in plain talk. These include addiction, depression, and anxiety. I explain the S.T.A.R. system and related concepts, such as healing the wounds of our past. I don't avoid issues other people may hide or feel embarrassed about. After reading and working your way through this book, you will find you don't have to either.

My practice is all about healing those parts of us that are wounded. Here you will discover the means to help you heal and deal with what went on in the past and the tools to equip you to go forward in your brand-new life.

This book and the S.T.A.R. system are for those of you who are ready to understand how life works. You are prepared to do the work to put your past behind you and then take off in full living color!

Chapter 1
My Story

"Finding yourself empowers you to experience life fully."
— *Dr. Wayne Dyer*

Why start this book with my own story? I want to share my journey because I've had many experiences that may be similar to your own search for your true self. If I can make big changes that alter my life, the odds are that you can do it too. I hope my story encourages you to find direction, answer the tough questions, and achieve your long-term dreams.

Later in this book, I'll describe the steps you can take to reach your goals. First, let me tell you a bit about my own story.

Over the years, I've opened myself up to new possibilities and taken chances. These steps put me on the path to freedom, although I experienced some difficulties and trials along the way. Eventually, I finally became the independent woman with a career that I love.

That's certainly not the direction I thought my life was headed in thirty years ago. I believed that my role was to marry and become a housewife and mother. The conflict between taking that path and taking the one that I wanted, coupled with my less than optimal relationships, was just too much. I felt pushed toward confusion, self-doubt, and loneliness.

At that time, I struggled in my life. My biggest personal crisis was triggered by the break-up of what appeared to be a promising, romantic relationship. I experienced an emotional, mental, and physical crash. I began my personal journey at that low point and had to realize that I was insecure and so unsure of myself. From there, I rebuilt my life to finally become a much more resilient person.

First, I took a look at my childhood and the automatic expectations that I'd become a good housewife and raise children. The idea of a mandated role for women in my community made me uncomfortable. I admired strong independent women. My problem was that I didn't know how to become that kind of woman.

As I grew older, I started developing my own ideas about life and this created an internal conflict between becoming the person you're expected to be versus becoming the person you really want to be. I learned later that this is often why many of us face struggles in life. At the time, this conflict left me feeling stuck and confused.

I struggled to figure out what direction I should go in. I believed that a women's role was to be married, **and** have children. All my friends and family were living up to that expectation. So, why hadn't I?

I moved to a large city, Vancouver B.C., so that I could live independently, find a job and sort things out. My problem? I was miserable in every job. I watched the clock and waited for Fridays. I felt lost, confused, and stuck in job after miserable job.

Nothing in my life was working — the jobs or my relationships with men. I felt unloved, rejected, and misunderstood.

Why couldn't I be like everyone else I knew? I believed that there must be something wrong with me. Why was my life so difficult? Why couldn't my life be just as easy as everyone else's?

One day, I decided to try something new. I applied for a retail job in a shopping mall and I was hired on the spot. Within a few days, I was working with people, merchandising clothing, setting up sales and listening to music whilst I worked. It was amazing! I realized I loved the job. I wasn't sitting at a desk all day in silence.

I learned I had far too much energy for that. I loved talking and interacting with people. It dawned on me that *I had been doing the wrong job*. Office work was what *I thought I should do*. Within six months, I was offered my own store as a manager.

What a difference! I loved my job and loved helping people.

The Beginning of the End

My life began to look more promising. I met a man, and I finally felt "normal." After a few years in a relationship with him, we began to talk about getting married. However, that was as far as it went. As the years went by, I wondered, "What's going on?" He claimed he wanted to marry me but he wasn't fully committed.

I was so confused with his behavior, saying one thing and yet doing another. I thought it must be my fault. I didn't want to give up on the relationship and leave him so, I chose to hang in there in complete misery hoping he would change and we would live happily ever after. Instead, the situation went downhill. His words didn't match his behavior and my head was spinning. There I was with a wedding dress and a ring on my finger. What the heck?? I then became suspicious that he was being unfaithful. It was easier to blame myself for being so insecure.

One day, his stepmother hesitantly told me that my fiancée had brought another woman to her house. When I heard that, I felt like I had been punched in the gut. My legs became weak, and my stomach was in my throat. I was horrified. I couldn't believe what I had just heard!

I phoned him and asked for an explanation. He claimed it was **my** fault.

I had thoughts like, "How terrible was I to push him into the arms of another woman?"

"I should try harder and be more loving."

"It must be me. I drove him away."

As the situation became worse, I wanted to see for myself what he was up to, in order to prove to myself that he wasn't deceiving me. I started going to the gym where he claimed he was going. I never saw him there. "Probably another lie!" I was somewhat relieved that I didn't catch him. In spite of not being able to reassure myself that he was telling me the truth, I did get something out of going to the gym… I was getting in fantastic shape.

Finally, I begged a mutual acquaintance to confirm my suspicions of him being with another girl so that I could come to terms with it and let go. As painful as it would be, I knew I had to move on from this constant mistrust in him and also the pain that I was in that was affecting me so deeply. As I had suspected, they confirmed that there was indeed another girl. I asked for her name and phone number just to prove to myself yet again that there was no mistake. I just didn't want to see what was so obvious. They gave me her details and I called her. We arranged to meet up the next day. She had no idea I existed.

She told me that he'd also promised to marry her. I was shocked and felt so damn stupid. We compared stories and she was surprised and disturbed by his behaviour. I couldn't continue to deny the truth. That's when I, finally, was able to completely let go emotionally! FINALLY!

That was it. Once I had freed myself from the denial I had been living in for years and recognized the toxicity of the relationship, I was then able to realize just how desperate and how **much** I was willing to put up with just to be with somebody!

As the months passed after the breakup, I was still confused about my life. I was 27 years old and single, which was frowned upon and very unusual where I came from. The relationship that was finally going to save me and make me look good in front of my family and friends. So where was I going to go from here?

I had been so sure that a relationship would make my life ideal. I thought that all I needed was to find the one, get married, have kids and that would be it. I would be happy and feel complete.

The old tapes of my childhood and *who I thought I should be* kept me stuck believing that this was the formula to happiness. Although the revelation of his cheating was painful, it also inspired me to change my life in powerful ways.

There was one thing I was certain about; *I was never going to go through anything like that again!* Something in me had to change.

My Healing

I wasn't sure where to start or where to turn. How do I change myself? I began to see a counselor and read lots of books on personal growth. I had been asking myself: How could I have let this happen? How could I let someone treat me this way? How did I let a relationship that wasn't working go on for so long? What was wrong with me? As I focused on myself and began to grow as a person, I started to find answers to these questions. It was time to make peace with myself and with my story.

I was so broken that I was unable to go to work for an entire year. During that year, I worked on my well-being exclusively. I took the time to focus on myself in order to enable the positive changes I knew were necessary and to heal the wounds that my experiences had left on my psyche. I wanted to feel in control of my life, be more confident, and have a sense of well-being.

Through counseling sessions and reading self-help books, I began to understand that my childhood and other experiences had created wounds that manifested themselves as self-doubt and feelings of inadequacy. I worked hard to heal and move on from my past.

The Transformation

I worked out at the gym, I wrote letters, and I kept a daily journal. As I worked on myself, I grew stronger emotionally and began to understand who I truly was. As my self-awareness and confidence grew, I began to notice that I was attracting attention from many types of men - professionals, athletes, younger and older – that I had never thought would be interested in me. This shocked me. *How wrong I had been to believe that I was unlovable and not good enough!* I began to date, but I never let myself become emotionally invested. I was vulnerable and fragile.

The shift came when I decided I was going to take charge of my life. I needed to choose between two opposite directions my life could go. One direction was the way I thought I was sup-posed to live my life and the type of woman I had been raised to believe I should be. The other direction was the dream I had for myself --what I really thought and felt I wanted. I really wanted to live my life as a confident, independent, self-assured and strong woman. This choice, between who you think you should be and who you truly desire to be, can be a major step for most people.

I made my choice. I was done trying to be and do what I had believed was expected. I wanted to become strong and self-assured. *And as for relationships, I wasn't going to wait for a man to decide if I was good enough for him. Instead, **I** was going to decide if **he** was good enough for **me**!!*

With this new confidence, I knew I was ready to get back to work.

Firstly, I was hired by a retail giant. A month into the job, my previous employer contacted me and offered me a manag-er's position. I accepted.

When I gave my notice, the management at the new job reacted quickly and offered me a managerial position in the menswear department. Wow! Here I was, after years of feeling rejected and "not good enough," now, suddenly people were fighting to keep me in their company, **and** men were knocking on my door. It is amazing how when…..you change the way you feel about yourself, people see you differently.

The Dream

One morning, a few years later, I awoke from a lucid dream about the Lions Gate Bridge. Lions Gate is a 1930's era suspen-sion bridge in Vancouver, BC that connects the downtown core to the mountainous North Shore. I was captivated by this dream.

I constantly wanted to go to the bridge. I would drive to Stanley Park and sit in my car and stare at the bridge. What was it about this bridge? Why was I so drawn to it? I wanted to touch it, be on it. If I saw a picture of the bridge, I felt butterflies in my stomach. It was an unexplainable fixation.

Then one day I decided I was going to walk across this bridge. I was convinced that if I walked across the bridge I would find the answer to "What's next in my life?"

I felt that on the other side of the bridge was the beginning of something new. I believed that once I reached the other side of that bridge, I would soon meet the man I would marry and I would enter the next phase of my life. A male friend offered to drive me to the Vancouver side so that I could walk to the North Shore side and back.

I began to walk across the bridge from one end to the other. I kept asking the questions, "What is it about this bridge? Is there something I need to know?" I reached the North Shore end and knew I wanted to cross over to the other sidewalk and then walk back over the bridge again, to where my friend was waiting for me. The traffic was moving fast and I wondered how I would cross to the other side and continue my journey. I looked around and there it was—an underpass to get to the other side! Wow! *If we stop and look around, there is always a way to get where we need to be.*

I continued to walk and jog across the massive bridge, asking the questions, "What is the message here?" Then the answer came. I heard my calling as clear as day: **"Take what you've learned, and teach it to others!"**

What happened to the friend who drove me to the Lions Gate Bridge, and who waited while I journeyed across and back? My premonition that I'd find the man I would marry at the end of the bridge came true! That friend has been my husband for over twenty years.

What I learned from my experience

- *Never doubt your gut feelings*

- *If you feel conflicted and struggle **continuously** with your situation, you probably **shouldn't be in that situation***

- *How you live your life today has **everything** to do with your past experiences, they are the lens through which you view the world*

- *When you struggle in life, look **inward***

- *Have the courage to **let go of the expectations** of the people you love in order to find yourself*

Chapter 2
You Can Heal

*"Happiness is not determined by what's happening around you,
but rather what's happening inside you. Most people depend
on others to gain happinessbut the truth is,
it always comes from within."*
-- Unknown

Introduction

In this chapter, you're going to explore some of the issues that the system in this book can help you with, and discover how to identify and trust your feelings. I learned from the experiences in 'My Story' and from those of my clients.

Feelings can be difficult and unpleasant. They can also be fantastic. Embracing life means that you're willing to deal with both the easy feelings and the hard feelings.

I urge you to never doubt your gut feelings. Also, I encourage you to take on problems like depression, anxiety, and addiction and learn to heal yourself with the right kind of self-exploration.

Trust your distress.
It tells you something is not right in your life.

If you're distressed in some way, sit up and pay attention. Maybe you've started to cry for no reason. Or you've become extremely worried about things you know aren't that important in the big picture. You may find yourself flying into a rage over a minor incident. You may have nagging thoughts that you're not acting or doing things the way you "should."

Are any of the examples below similar to how you feel?

- I feel anxious and fearful.
- I am a people pleaser.
- I am a rebel.
- I feel there is something wrong with me.
- I feel guilty if I don't put others' needs before mine.
- I am rigid and a perfectionist. I am driven to be a super achiever.
- I feel empty most of the time.
- I am angry.
- I feel ashamed of myself.
- I am afraid to be alone.
- I am very sensitive about what others think about me or what they say.
- I am sad/depressed.
- I am addicted to alcohol, drugs, cigarettes, food, shopping, gaming, and social media.
- I struggle in relationships.
- I am lazy.
- I'm not motivated.
- I don't know what I want.
- I don't fit in socially. I stay away from people.

Your feelings are a gauge. Accept and trust them.

Observe and take note of your feelings. Welcome them. Use them to gauge how well you're doing.

Consider some of these questions.

Do you feel?

- Rejected by your partner?
- Angry at a situation?
- Hurt because you feel you've disappointed someone or someone disappointed you?
- Stressed from your job?

You may be experiencing feelings like these and choosing to ignore them or you may be unaware of how these feelings may be affecting you. Instead, you may reach for the outside answer to provide quick relief from what you feel.

It's important to accept all your feelings, good and bad. They're just feelings. They come and go, and at times are unpredictable, but everyone has them. Trust those core feelings. They're your compass in life and will steer you true. Focus on what you *feel* to have a better understanding of what's going on in your life.

Whatever the reason is for the turmoil you feel, it's important to *trust your gut*. Why? Because your gut feelings tell you that something in your life isn't working.

If you feel pulled every which way and feel that your life is difficult, take a close look at your social, home and work situations. You may be able to identify the cause of your turmoil. Once you know your own distress signals, it's time to find out what's going on. But where do you look? As you work through the system outlined in this book, you will discover that the answers are available to you, with introspection and work.

Are you depressed or anxious?

Depression and anxiety can be signs of feelings that you are unaware of, a story that needs to be told. You may need to talk about these feelings and work through them.

Anxiety symptoms include not feeling safe or feeling like you have to stay one step ahead. You fear that if you don't stay ahead you will fall apart, spiral out of control, or *something* bad will happen. You could also feel overwhelmed with responsibilities. You may have had a traumatic experience and are experiencing the feelings of that trauma on a regular basis. Perhaps you've been diagnosed as having anxiety or depression. If you've been given a diagnosis or label like this, it may not be a life sentence.

I believe that it is possible to overcome anxiety, depression, and addiction by looking at your past and current experiences and how they influence the way you live. Then work to heal the wounds from your past that you have left unexplored. In my experience working with clients, I have seen a very positive response to this kind of therapy.

Addiction is basically a way to avoid difficult, uncomfortable emotions or an effort to achieve an emotion. For many, addiction can be a sign of poor coping skills.

Addiction is a problem that is usually the result of a strong, uncomfortable feeling. You might feel sad, hurt, frustrated, or miserable about yourself, and try to feel better. Yes, you may have a genetic predisposition to addiction. Several factors can contribute to addictive tendencies. However, you can overcome that inclination with hard work and dedication.

Often, the set up for addiction or addictive behaviour is the thought, "Get me out of this feeling," or "Get me into a better feeling." The underlying belief may be, "I'm not good enough,

I hate the way I feel. I don't want to remember what happened to me."

People who struggle with addiction or negative behaviour will try to find something to change their mood. They look for a quick fix to escape their current thoughts and feelings. The majority of them seek emotional numbness. Ending addiction can be difficult because the withdrawal from a substance can cause pain and make you very sick. You may be physically addicted as well as mentally and emotionally addicted.

Maybe you hope something will come along that makes you feel less empty. You may find relief by turning to alcohol, cigarettes, or any type of drug or addictive behaviour that "works" temporarily. Did you know that addictive behaviours also include overeating, overworking, trying to please everyone, shopping, and gambling? Ultimately, these attempts to feel better fail to solve anything.

Stop and listen to your inner voice. Be in the moment and pay attention! What's going on inside of you every time you decide that it's time to pick up a drink or smoke a cigarette? Or when you go out and spend money on things you don't really need? Ask yourself, "What am I trying to avoid? Is it a feeling or a negative voice inside my head?"

Something or someone has caused you to believe negative thoughts about yourself. You need to acknowledge and heal those places that have been wounded. These are the underlying issues that make you feel things you are trying to avoid. Getting "high" or engaging in an addictive behaviour won't solve the fact that you feel badly about yourself. When you change how you cope with uncomfortable feelings, you also propel change in your addictive behaviour.

One of the reasons our society is so addicted is because many of us were never taught to deal with our feelings. Developing good coping skills is a must if you come from a family with addiction or if your parents never healed their wounds. If you weren't allowed to talk about or express your feelings, then the odds are high that you could become an addict or develop a behaviour that hurts you. When you develop healthy coping skills and can recognize what causes you to turn to your addiction, you receive the key to a life of sobriety and emotional well-being.

Understanding your feelings doesn't necessarily resolve your problem. It's not always enough to move you into a healthier state. For example, you know that your addictive behaviour hurts you and the people around you but you can't stop it. You often deal with both the emotional and the physical symptoms of addiction.

Your addiction maybe destroying your life. You might be losing your family because of the addiction, problems at work, possibly even financial destruction. So why is it so hard to stop?

It's more than dealing with cravings. It is important to acknowledge and work through the strong emotions that could be keeping you stuck. When you address and heal the unresolved emotional issues, it is possible to move forward in a more positive direction.

Healing comes from the deepest part of your soul. It has to resonate through your whole body, not just in your head. Reading or talking about change can give you a deeper understanding of what is going on for you. If you want fundamental change, then you must heal and recover from your past.

You can heal the wounds

'Heal' has a few definitions. It means, 'to restore to health', or 'to ease or relieve emotional distress', or 'to set right or repair.' All three of these definitions can apply when we talk about healing the wounds of the past.

You may feel helpless and hopeless about what happened to you. You may not be happy about where you are at in your life. Or you feel that there just isn't any clear path to resolve these feelings. I'm telling you that there is.

Whether this is your first self-help book or if you've read many, you're searching for something better in your life and you're looking for answers. I hope that this book gives you a deeper understanding of how we work as humans, and how you can regain a sense of self-worth.

You're worthy because you're alive … that's it …

When you take action, you'll find that success and lasting change are much easier to achieve. You will be able to deal with your underlying issues. We operate from the subconscious mind – the storage room of everything that's currently not in your conscious mind. The subconscious mind is where we carry our thoughts of ourselves, our beliefs, and our unexplained choices.

We are all logical beings. When we find ourselves giving in to a negative behaviour or we keep making bad choices, this may indicate that the subconscious is taking charge and is strong and alive within us. Our underlying issues are strong and alive.

Where you were wounded, the subconscious mind is the place you live your life from!

Move toward self-reliance and happiness

Dealing with past hurt, trauma, or abuse is a process. Take your time, work through your feelings slowly. There is no quick recovery from your past. I will offer some suggestions on how to deal with this pain, how to release it in a structured way so that you can heal.

At the end of 'My Story', I wrote: "How you live your life today has everything to do with your past experiences." What happened to you in your past has shaped the person that you are today. It created the patterns in your behaviours and the thoughts that you have about yourself. The things that occurred in your past impact your choices in the present. When bad things happened to you, you may have found ways to protect yourself, ways that might not be helping you in your life today.

Just know that **you can change your life**. Take the time to rediscover your life and your experiences so that you can get a clear picture of what contributed to the person you are today. In the next chapter, you'll read about the system that I use in my counseling practice. The work you have done in this chapter to identify the issues you are facing has laid the groundwork for you to use the steps I have identified to improve your life.

Chapter 3
The STAR System

"Courage is never to let your actions be influenced by your fears."
-- Arthur Koestler

As a professional counsellor, I have supported and witnessed some amazing personal transformations and successes. In this chapter, you will read about my special brand of therapy, which I call the STAR system.

The S.T.A.R. system is shorthand for the principles that underlie most of my work. Following these principles can help you change your life from confusion, helplessness or hopelessness to one of happiness, fulfillment and satisfaction.

These principles are:

S = Self-reliance

T = Transformation

A = Action

R = Results

You are probably wondering what each of these terms mean. In this chapter, you will read an overview of each principle.

'S' Stands for Self-Reliance

Self-reliance starts with taking responsibility for yourself emotionally, physically, and mentally in a completely honest way. Make sure you have a clear idea of where you are going and know what kind of life you want. Think about what your values are and set some definite boundaries. It is important that **you** make the decisions about your life.

Afraid? Move *towards* your fears, not away from them. If you really want something, you're going to have to do whatever it takes to move past the fear of change or the fear of looking deep inside the places that you may have tried to get past. Fear can keep you from moving forward and becoming the person you really want to be. Usually, fear comes from a negative experience.

Fear keeps us safe. However, needing to stay safe in all aspects of your life will keep you from growing and living the life you want.

If you were bullied as a child, you may avoid going to places or functions where there are people you don't know. When we are faced with a situation that brings back a negative memory, we may try to avoid it. If you fell off your bike several times, you may avoid riding a bike. Whatever the negative experience is that we had, we attach fear to it and attempt to avoid similar situations.

Change happens when we let go of the negative experiences and look to the future with a new attitude. You may have had a bad experience doing something. That doesn't mean you will have the same experience every time. So, you've fallen off your bike several times. You aren't necessarily going to fall off your bike every time you try to ride it.

Remember, you're the one who has to change.

Accept what is—but if you can't accept it, change it.

Stop blaming others for the way you feel. You probably already feel that way, but you just haven't acknowledged it. When someone makes a comment that hits you in the gut, ask yourself, "Is this true? Do I feel this way about myself? Do I agree with what was said?" If you answer "Yes" to either of those questions, acknowledge it first. Then, begin to look at why you were affected so deeply. It is one thing to feel a little hurt or disturbed by someone's words or disapproval of you. It's another thing when it takes over your life. What is your reason for agreeing with the negative or hurtful thing that was said to you?

Love for yourself shouldn't come from others' approval and acceptance of you. It cannot come from anything external. Loving yourself comes from your *own* approval and acceptance.

That is what self-reliance is -- learning to love yourself. You don't have to rely on anyone but yourself to meet your emotional needs.

'T' is for Transformation

Transformation requires you to take responsibility for what you feel and think. What is being transformed is the way you think about yourself. Instead of looking for someone else's approval or acceptance, you are able to approve of and accept yourself.

Transformation occurs when you understand *who you are,* including how you think and act. The central core of you is more important than:

What you do for work or for "status." We often wrap ourselves in this exterior label to show the world that we are "good and successful."

Or, you may be focused on......

What you have. This includes your possessions, the balance of your bank account, all of the material things that society tells us we need to have in order to be important. You define yourself this way.

Transformation takes place when you begin to live the life you want, not the life you think you "should" live based on someone else's perception or the life someone else has said you should live. It is necessary to work through the negative experiences in your past, in order to **transform** the way you manage your life and manage the memories you have. Later in the book, we'll look at some ways to help you work through these experiences.

It is important to see the world as cause and effect. The respect you show yourself will be in line with the respect you give to others and the respect you receive from others. This occurs because when you respect yourself, you will not tolerate disrespect from others. You teach people how to treat you.

Transformation is a process. By working on understanding your emotions, you begin to understand how and why you have been affected by your past and why you react the way you do in the present.

'A' is for Action

You must take action to see results. If you've decided you want a different life and it's time to change, then you must start to make different choices.

Once you know the specific differences you would like to see in your life, decide the direction you need to take to get there. This can be a big task.

Here are some suggestions that will help you focus on your goal of making change in your life:

- Take small steps that progress toward that bigger goal.
- If you have too many goals, focus on one at a time.
- Write each goal down as clearly as you can.
- Break each goal down by mapping out the steps to achieve it.

Include focused and concrete actions in your goal map. Then, start to carry out your plan. Take daily action, even if it's only small steps toward the goal you're working to achieve.

What you do means much more than what you say, Action is a catalyst for change.

Do something *every* day to move toward your goals. Action will produce results!

'R' is for Results

Once you've followed these steps, you'll make choices that genuinely reflect your true self and fulfill your needs.

When you engage with life in this positive, proactive way, you'll find happiness. And even better news…..This joyful journey will continue on and on.

Conclusion

Hopefully when you finish reading this book, the S.T.A.R. system will have gone from being words to being a system you thoroughly understand at a deep level. In the next chapter, you'll explore the concept of self-reliance more thoroughly.

Chapter 4
Our Basic Needs

"Peace comes from within, do not seek it without."
– Bhudda

As you learn more about what makes you tick, you will become increasingly confident and independent. Self-reliance is based in understanding and fulfilling your physical, emotional, and spiritual needs for yourself. You don't have to look to anyone else to do it for you. What are the steps you need to take? That is what this chapter addresses.

Physical needs

Physically, each of us requires food, water, shelter, and sleep. Eating nutritiously, drinking enough fluids, maintaining a place to live, and getting enough sleep are the ways that we meet our physical needs.

Emotional Needs

Emotionally, we all need to feel good and to feel valued, loved, supported and worthy. One way we do this is to seek companionship and connectedness. Meeting our emotional needs is about trusting our feelings to let us know what we need, when we need it. It is not as straightforward as meeting our physical needs.

Let's focus on how we identify and meet our emotional needs. We should first understand what emotions are.

What is Emotion?

Emotional energy is energy that moves. Emotion carries the entire spectrum of feelings. Understanding that *emotions are energy* implies that they are fluid, moving resources. Emotions are meant to be felt, and released not suppressed and ignored.

It is important to move your emotions by recognizing them, expressing them, and talking to someone about them. It is generally easy to do this with positive emotions because we want to share and celebrate positive emotions.

It can be more difficult with negative emotions such as fear, sadness, grief, guilt, and shame. If you don't acknowledge your negative emotions, they can become stuck and may emerge as stress, depression, anxiety, addiction, or unhealthy behaviour. Your emotions tell you what you need to do, what you want, or what you need to change.

Everyone experiences emotional turbulence at times. By keeping a daily journal, you will be able to recognize, express and acknowledge the emotions that lie deep inside you and the needs they present. Recognizing these helps you to function as a healthier happier human being. You will find certain emotions will wax and wane and that you are often in a state of flux. So, keep on your toes and be ready to deal with whatever comes up.

When you feel sad, allow yourself the time to connect to the feeling. Examine it and attempt to discover the source of the sadness and then allow the feeling to pass. Fighting the feeling may keep you from understanding what the sadness is about for you.

Sometimes just picking up your journal and jotting some thoughts down as you feel sad will give you an insight into what brought up the emotion. Feeling your emotions is important. We are emotional beings. Feelings tell us what's wrong, what's not working for us, and that we're frightened or sad. They can also tell us we are happy and on the right track.

The negative emotions are important signposts that tell us that some emotional need is not being met. You need to allow yourself time to explore these negative emotions. They are the emotions that most people are afraid of, yet they are the most important ones to recognize to ensure that our emotional needs are met.

Experiencing negative emotions sometimes means that something needs to change in our lives. Other times, such as when we are sad about losing a loved one, we just need to accept that the emotions are there, and that there is nothing wrong with feeling them. The simple act of acknowledging the existence of a feeling may be all that is needed.

Spiritual Needs

Spirituality has a different meaning for each of us. Generally, when you include spirituality in your healing process, you open yourself to a larger perspective. You value yourself and see value in others and in all forms of life. You start to realize that everyone has difficulties; that everyone has their own struggles to deal with. This perspective can help you become a more caring and kinder person.

It can also help you appreciate your own value in the larger scheme of things. You begin to recognize that your past experiences may have prepared you to help someone else, to change the lives of those around you in some way. My difficult experiences, and the growth that I had to go through, have allowed me to better connect with and help my clients. Each of us has a personal sense of our soul. Satisfy your personal needs around your own beliefs.

Understanding your emotional needs is the key to self-reliance

Your physical, emotional, and spiritual needs will change over time. Understanding what they are and the healthiest way to fulfill them is part of everyone's journey. With emotional self-reliance comes a certain amount of stability.

You will no longer feel powerless and lost as a result of a stressful life event. For example, your partner may leave you. You may feel upset, angry, and sad. It's natural to feel this way. However, you will be confident that you will be okay in the end. You have weathered storms before and you will weather them again.

If you haven't healed your past hurts and pain, a stressful event such as your partner leaving, could lead to anxiety, depression, or even manifest as addiction to help you cope. This healing of your past pain will allow you to become much more emotionally self-reliant. Until these hurts are healed, accepted, forgiven or viewed differently, they will continue to impact the way you view yourself, and also the way you react to situations in the present.

We are forever learning about ourselves and growing

When you work through an issue, it makes your future challenges easier to bear. You must remain self-aware.

You may be surprised by the significant improvements you are able to make in your life. However, a day may come when you feel like you are back in another dark place. This could mean that you have more work to do!

You have many layers, just like an onion. You may peel back the outer layers, feel fantastic, go out there, and enjoy life. Then other issues might start to arise. We each learn and grow throughout our life, and it all starts with understanding yourself.

How to increase your emotional self-reliance

Know your values

Values help you understand what you need. You will make better decisions if you follow your moral code. If you believe that you value honesty, ask yourself "Am I being honest with myself and others?" If the answer is "Yes" then you are in line with your values.

- Is your life in line with your values?
- Does your life currently reflect your values?
- Are your values consistent with your actual behaviour?
- What kind of changes would you need to make to keep yourself in line with your personal values?

Example   Let us assume that you value kindness. If you behave in a way that is unkind towards others, or you allow others to treat you unkindly, you are not living in line with your values. This leads to a sense that you are off balance in your life.

Perhaps you believe that you value family. However, you spend all of your time at work, or busy with other things. You don't spend much time with your family. This behaviour does not align with your claim that you value family.

To truly value family, you must live it. Change your life to place more importance on spending quality time with your family. Then you can see that your behaviours and values line up. This will make you feel more centered and balanced.

Define your boundaries

Defining your boundaries is an important part of the whole process. You will begin to understand who you are and what types of behavior or thoughts affect you more than others.

If you feel uncomfortable in a situation, it can often be an indication that your boundaries have been crossed. You may need to reinforce your boundaries.

For example, what do you do when someone talks to you in a way that makes you feel uncomfortable?

You can say, "I'm not comfortable with this conversation," and walk away.

Boundaries are about what's *not* okay with you. They are guidelines, rules, or limits that you create for yourself.

Your boundaries identify what are reasonable and permissible ways for others to behave around you. Boundaries let you know when someone steps outside those limits and it is time for you to respond. There are several types of boundaries. They include:

Material boundaries help you determine if you are willing to give or lend things. For example, whether or not you are willing to loan a friend your car, your favorite shoes, or money.

Physical boundaries involve your personal space, privacy and body. For example, whether or not you allow anyone to physically touch you.

Mental boundaries concern your thoughts, values and opinions. For example, if you are willing to let your partner read your journal, or if you are going to allow yourself to be talked into doing something that makes you uncomfortable.

Emotional boundaries have to do with your ability to separate your emotions and responsibilities from anyone else's. Having healthy emotional boundaries can help you to avoid taking someone's comment personally.

They can also help you to not feel responsible for and guilty about someone else's negative emotions or problems.

For example, your partner is upset about having been late for work and blames you. However, your partner had slept in, and you had already left for work by the time he or she had intended to wake up.

If you have healthy emotional boundaries, instead of accepting that blame, you can recognize that your partner's problem is not your fault and you have no reason to feel guilty or responsible.

You have to be clear about what your boundaries are. If something is going on that is not acceptable to you, and you keep allowing it, ask yourself, "Why am I allowing this?" Say what you are thinking. "This is my boundary. This is not acceptable to me."

If you continue to allow people to cross boundaries that you have set for yourself, you may begin to feel helpless and unhappy. When you stand firm with your boundaries, you teach people how to treat you. If you don't let others know right away when they say something, or behave in a way that is unacceptable to you, they will continue with their behaviour. You will be miserable.

Strong boundaries are closely related to a strong self-esteem and self-respect. Once you start practicing boundaries, you start building your self-respect.

If standing up for yourself is difficult, you may feel helpless or feel you don't have a right to stand up for yourself. This feeling could have been created very early in your life. If you don't heal and move past your childhood trauma and abuse, you may remain stuck believing that this is just the way it is.

It is your responsibility to protect yourself from anything that you know will hurt you. As a child, you looked to mom and dad to stand up for you and take care of you. That was their job then. Now that you are an adult, it is your job to take care of yourself.

"Your tormentor of today is your past left over from yesterday."
-- Deepak Chopra

Notice what you like about people.

It tells you something about the type of person you want to be. A good question to ask is *"What do I see, and look up to in other people that make me wish I was more like them?"*

All of us look to certain people. Although you may not know why at first, usually you will recognize something about that person that you would like to cultivate in yourself.

Accept support from others

Look at yourself as the *primary* foundation. Secondary assistance also helps. Keep in mind everyone needs help from other people. Reach out.

Some people find it helps to have a mentor. There are many kinds of mentors, and not all of them are official.

If you've taken a work-related course at a community college and really clicked with the instructor, he or she might make a good career mentor for you.

Perhaps you get regular massages from a massage therapist and admire her calm outlook. Share a minor issue with her and see if she offers an insight. Many people in this type of occupation have pursued their own personal growth and have wisdom to share.

Counselling is another option to consider. A therapist can help reinforce the positive moves in your life and help you through turbulent times if you feel stuck. They can also help you address your past and help you understand how it affects you today so you can make a different choice based on this new understanding.

You can find structured and unstructured support in many places. A sponsor from a 12-step program and a leader in your religious community are examples of those who offer structured support.

Less formal support can come from friends and family members. Search for like-minded men and women who can guide you.

Associate with people who you feel are growing and learning. It's not wise to choose those who struggle with serious issues in their own lives. They may not have the strength or know how to support you in a healthy way.

Instead, look for mutually supportive friendships. Make sure you are on equal footing with your friends.

And remember; trust *yourself to* know what has to change.

Conclusion

Remember to take care of your physical, emotional, and spiritual needs.

Keep in mind emotions are constantly in motion and that every feeling will fade and be replaced with another as time passes.

Personal values are an important part of the puzzle. Take the time to figure out what *you* think is right and wrong. It is important. When you understand your values, it is easier to set firm and clear boundaries with others. When you feel hurt by someone's behaviour, you will quickly arrive at an understanding of what is going on for you and stop accepting what doesn't feel right for you.

Change can be a positive, active process. Notice those around you, what you dislike, *and especially what traits you admire.* Pay attention to the people you like most.

Accept support from others. Being self-reliant doesn't mean you have to do everything by yourself all of the time. It means that you should look to yourself to understand and fulfill your needs first.

Everyone needs support sometimes, but it is important not to rely on anyone but yourself to meet your needs.

Now that you know what self-reliance is and have discovered some ways to increase your self-reliance, it is time to dig into your life and find the experiences in your past that still hurt you.

Negative past experiences can cause us pain in the present. They influence the way we think about ourselves, the way we think about others, and our perception of our experiences.

Next, you will investigate your life, to find these negative experiences and how they impact your life today.

Chapter 5
Investigate Your Life

"I am who I am today, because of the choices I made yesterday."
—Eleanor Roosevelt

Now it is time to explore your life and take a closer look at yourself. Don't tense up! You can do it. You've read this far. I know you have the courage to continue. Progress at your own pace and ask for help if you need it.

Try to approach this with an attitude of curiosity and be open to what you might discover. As you collect clues like the forensic specialists on the television show *CSI* (aka Crime Scene Investigation), this is your chance to become a sleuth. Seek the details. Watch for red herrings. Clues will turn up in both expected *and* unexpected places.

Investigate your life

One of the best methods to collect these clues is to jot down your thoughts in a daily journal. Set aside at least ten minutes each day to enter some of your reflections on the day.

Some observations to note in your journal:

- Identify when you have strong feelings.
- What are the circumstances?
- Where are you?
- What time of day is it?
- Are you alone or with other people?
- What are the thoughts going on in your mind?
- Did someone say something that changed the way you feel?

Focus particularly on thoughts that repeat again and again like 'broken tapes.' Write about your positive emotions, like satisfaction, pleasure, and joy. Also, write about your negative emotions, like sadness, fear, and anger.

You will start to notice that specific things 'trigger' you. By this, I mean that certain things tend to precede a particular emotion. These things are potentially a cause of the emotion, or make you more likely to experience that emotion. Triggers can be just about anything — an image, a smell, a taste, or someone else's behaviour.

Triggers cause you to have an intense emotional reaction. When you start to examine them, you will see that negative emotions may often be triggered by an unresolved event from your past. The trigger has brought the emotions to the surface of your subconscious. This reaction seems similar to post traumatic stress disorder (PSTD).

Here is an example of being triggered:-

"My husband just told me I'm incompetent. I remember that my dad used to tell me that I couldn't do anything right when I was growing up. I'd storm out of the house and go to the nearby shopping mall and spend hours trying on clothes until I calmed down. I'm doing the same thing now … I didn't know that was a trigger for me. When I would feel hurt and feel I had failed, I would go out and compulsively shop for clothes… Now I realize what's going on!"

When you understand what's behind your unhelpful or destructive actions, it enables you to stop repeating them. When you are conscious of the trigger, it may no longer have the ability to ambush you and cause you to take action that may be unnecessary. The memory becomes just an experience you had. Its power over you is gone. Try to become more conscious and pay attention to how you feel. Understanding your triggers may not be enough to stop the behavior or the choices you make but it is a good start.

Investigate your life. The evidence is inside you. When a comment cuts you to the core, you know that it is more than a mean comment because it really set off something deeper in you. For example, your inner voice will tell you, "People are always mean to me" or "I'm just not good enough."

Try to become mindful of your inner voice. Pay attention to the negative self-chatter that keeps you in an unpleasant place. If you constantly feel upset about people's comments and behaviour, it is time to make some changes. It may help if you focus on building your confidence and self-esteem.

When you realize how your childhood, your school years, your parents, and your teachers may have negatively affected you, you gain new insight. You suddenly understand why certain situations repeatedly make you act in a predictable way.

This new insight will help you find the clues to why you may feel depressed, why all of a sudden you feel anxious, why in a flash you go into a rage, or why you shut down emotionally. These changes occur because that part of you has not healed yet or you have not acknowledged the triggering event yet. You have work to do before the healing can occur.

You can't change what you don't first acknowledge. *The only way out is through.*

You may have had one of these difficult experiences in the past:

- You lived in a toxic family who constantly fought, name-called, and had inconsistent rules.
- You were told or felt that you weren't good enough.
- You struggled in school.
- You were bullied by your peers.
- You did not know your mother or father.
- Your parents were not there for you when you needed them.
- Nobody talked about his or her feelings in the family.
- Your parents, one or both of them, had an addiction.

Clients often tell me that their upbringing was good. Mom and Dad were there and everything was normal. However, normal looks different to all of us. What seems normal to you is not always healthy.

A child who was spanked when he said "No" or did something the parent did not agree with, may say that getting a spanking when mom or dad were unhappy was normal.

If you grew up in an alcoholic family, you may say that being around people who drink excessively is normal. However, this behaviour may have had a negative effect on you. Can you relate to any of the situations above or do you have any long-held negative beliefs about yourself? You may have had experiences that have affected the way you see yourself and how you see the world.

Where did you get derailed in life?
When did you lose yourself?

As you begin to trust and connect with your feelings, you will be able to look back and identify when things started to go wrong for you. This may have been in your early childhood or during your school years. In some cases, it may have been during young adulthood or mature adulthood. Childhood is where you were set up for life.

You learned how life works from your mother and father. You witnessed how they related to each other and to you. You also saw how they dealt with life's challenges. This experience can influence how you relate to others. It also may have impacted the way you see yourself and how you see the world. Your family taught you how to go through life. Their morals, views, opinions, and behaviours may have instructed you on how to face the world.

If a parent was never happy with your accomplishments and successes, it may have set you up with feelings of "I'm not good enough." It may have manifested as you becoming a perfectionist. You might feel like you need to do more and be more. Or you may be the polar opposite. You may have given up on yourself and do nothing at all.

What if your Mom or Dad drank an alcoholic beverage to relax or unwind after a day at work or when faced with a challenge? This may have set you up to use alcohol or drugs for the same reasons. If your parents didn't have good coping strategies, you may not have developed good coping skills yourself.

Learn how to take a step back, see where you were derailed in life, or where you were wounded and connect with that difficult time.

If this is too difficult, or if you feel like you just can't go there, please don't. You can get help with bringing these feelings and memories out with a trained professional.

However, when you are ready, it is important that you confront your feelings about the negative issues that are affecting you now. You must confront and work through those difficult times so that you can begin to move forward. It is important to understand that you do not have to do this alone. Talk to a therapist, counsellor, or a psychologist to get help and support.

All human pain is the same. It's the story that's different.

What does a dysfunctional family look like?

Here are a few examples of ways a family can be dysfunctional:

- Rigid gender based roles
- Approval must be earned
- Perfectionism
- Unexpressed or unacknowledged feelings
- Shaming/blaming
- Secrets - don't talk, don't tell rules
- Rigid family boundary
- Addiction
- Delusion/denial
- Control
- Unreliability
- Confusion
- Chronic anxiety/depression

Here are some traits of a family that functions in a healthy way:

- Parents who do what they say and who are reliable
- Family members can get their emotional needs met
- Family members are allowed to be different
- Communication is direct and congruent
- Family members can express feelings, thoughts, and desires
- Parents are flexible
- Family life is fun and comfortable
- The family members are accountable
- Mistakes are accepted and used to learn from and are forgiven
- Parents are in touch with their own needs and desires and don't look for their children to fulfill them.

If you realize your family could be dysfunctional, keep in mind that *every* family is dysfunctional at some level. No one knows how to be that 100% perfect family unit. We all come from what we know, that includes mom and dad.

You may find this fact healing. If your parents or a parent treated you badly by name-calling, put downs or never being there for you when you needed them, it wasn't because you are a bad person or didn't deserve better. Your parents just did what they knew and their behavior may have come from their own pain and fear. Possibly someone had treated them the same way in their past.

Parenting behaviours are passed from generation to generation. What could get passed on are feelings of "I'm not enough", or "I'm not good enough" and "I don't deserve love and kindness." If you didn't feel good enough for mom and dad or feel like you let your parents down, you may internalize this belief and carry it with you for a long while. As children, we look to our parents for approval and in some cases, we continue to look for our parent approval in adulthood.

What I hear quite often is, "But I do believe I deserve better." If that's the case, and you truly believe it, why would you be putting up with unsatisfactory behaviours and disrespect from others? Knowing isn't the same as truly believing it at every level of your being. When you truly believe it, your thoughts match your behaviour.

Our brain is logical. However, when we get our feelings hurt or when we are angry, all logic can go out the window. Our logic comes from the conscious level. When we say we know something, it also comes from this level. Our unresolved negative emotions come from the subconscious level, which can often contradict or override the logical conscious mind. This happens especially when we are feeling something deeply or when faced with a situation that touches a long-held subconscious belief.

This is why healing your past hurts and pain is so important. If you don't heal the past, it will continue to come up and make your life difficult. Once you understand these two concepts you are ready to move forward.

<u>Stop</u> looking for something or someone to make it right for you.

You may hope that someone or something will come along that will make everything "better." This type of thinking perpetuates an unhealthy pattern. You have all the resources inside and around you. You can draw on them to help you get better. Do as much of the internal work as you can. As I mentioned previously, you can also work with a trained professional to assure some extra support and direction as you make some important changes.

For example, let us say you hope that sometime soon your parents will finally recognize your achievements and acknowledge you for who you are and approve of your choices in life. Or maybe you just hope that they take some responsibility for their role in the way you see life or how you feel about yourself.

In some cases your parents may never say a word. This isn't because your parents are blind to your virtues or do not want to praise you or give you what you need. Your parents were unable to meet your needs because they did not understand what those needs were or they were not in a healthy place within themselves. *You can't give what you don't have!* If you don't have unconditional love, understanding and acceptance of yourself, you cannot give it to someone else. Eventually, you may begin to see your parents, your relationships and maybe even yourself with a new understanding.

Abuse or neglect is never acceptable. However, family dynamics are often repeated from generation to generation. You can understand that your parents may not have given you what you needed because they did not receive that praise, encouragement, and support either. What happens if your parents do not fulfill your emotional needs by offering unconditional love, structure, and praise for just being you? You may keep looking for someone or something to fulfill those needs.

You might want to stop seeking validation from your family and/or others. You can begin by asking yourself, "What is it that I needed and didn't get? Acceptance, love, attention, and praise?

Realize that we should not depend on others to validate who we are. It is nice but it is important not to depend on other people to make us feel better about ourselves. We should accept that we have all of the qualities that we are asking everyone else to recognize and praise. Most importantly, we are the ones who should acknowledge and praise them in ourselves.

If you continue to believe that your emotional well-being comes from someone else, you are not being emotionally self-reliant. You may not be accepting of the good qualities that you have. This denial keeps you safe and stuck to what you know right now. It insulates you from the hurt you may feel when you realize that you should have received praise as a child, but didn't. Denial can stop any growth and change from occurring in your life. Denial also impedes your ability to be emotionally self-reliant. If you look for someone else to give you value, it is because you are not giving yourself value. Recognizing your value is a key component of emotional self-reliance.

Our society encourages finding an "instant fix." However, achieving personal growth and awareness does not occur instantly. Look at your life, your patterns, and your story. Be an observer as well as a participant. You may need to work through many parts of your life.

You think, feel, and behave the way you do today, because of your family, social environment, and your positive and negative experiences.

Your biggest influences were your parents who were the number one role models in your life as you grew up. If you didn't observe good behaviour patterns and healthy ways to cope in stressful situations from your parents, you may struggle with feelings of confusion, self-doubt, and low self-esteem.

How your parents handled stress, how they communicated, how they dealt with their feelings and pain may have influenced how you handle yourself and how you behave.

Even if they never shared their past with you, your parents' behaviour influenced you.

If your parents' relationship was difficult, your chance of having healthy relationships and a positive outlook as an adult may be an uphill battle.

If your parents are unaware of their own emotional pain and how to express their feelings, they may not have been good role models for you. Children learn who they are and connect to their emotions through their parents. Learning to express and nurture feelings is healthy and necessary.

How you were raised wasn't about who you were. It was more about what your parents knew and how they felt about themselves.

Your childhood may have been painful. However, now you have the ability to change the legacy and do something different for yourself.

We all like to believe we have good values. A parent who spanks their child thinks that is the way to discipline. It is probably what he or she was taught in childhood. We now know that this kind of physical punishment may contribute to psychological and emotional difficulties in children all through their development and into their adulthood. The troubling results may be apparent immediately, or they may emerge years later.

Authority figures in your formative years may have affected your emotional and mental development. Usually your parent, teacher, or sports coach affected you either positively or negatively.

For example, children who have learning difficulties or are bullied in school can be horribly shamed. Children can carry that shame with them forever. They may begin to believe they are flawed, defective, and not as good or as smart as the other kids.

Conclusion

Be a detective and look at your own life. What are your triggers? Find out what is behind those triggers.

Remember that expecting others to fill your needs is only a temporary solution. Long-lasting change will only come when you do the work, heal, and grieve your past. It is only through mourning that we can begin to free ourselves from our past.

Many of the patterns in your life spring from repetitive past events. Triggers can create similar emotions today. Remember 'My Story' from the beginning of the book and what I learned from my experience. How you live your life and what affects you today is linked to your experiences in childhood and to your parents' unhealthy behaviors.

When you understand that people tend to see life and react to life's experiences based on their past, you will be able to free yourself from many unhealthy patterns.

As you peel away the layers and begin to understand yourself, your self-reliance and self-confidence will grow.

The skills you are learning here and the growth you are working on now are part of a lifelong journey. You will soon find there is *always* another layer you can discover!

If any of these examples or suggestions here have triggered emotions for you. Stay the course.

Next, you will discover how to heal the pain your past may be causing you.

Chapter 6
Begin to Heal Yourself

*"You gain strength, courage, and confidence
by every experience in which you really stop to
look fear in the face.
You must do the thing which you think you cannot do."*
--Eleanor Roosevelt

Introduction

In the last chapter, you investigated your life to find the hurts from your past. Now you will explore some ways to heal these hurts, to help you move forward. We will focus on self-reliance and transformation. You have learned what self-reliance is, have discovered some ways to increase your emotional self-reliance and have taken the steps of discovering your past pain.

Now it is time to transform the way you think about yourself and your past experiences. By using your newfound skills in emotional self-reliance, you have identified your emotional need to heal the pain that you carry from your past. For you to be in control of your emotions, you need to transform the way you think about your past experiences, and alter the way you think about yourself.

How do you heal?

You have explored your past to discover where you were derailed or wounded. Now it is time to face this time in your life. Pain from your past is like a splinter that broke off deep inside of you and has been festering. It often causes pain that may seem unrelated to the initial splinter, yet it is not. In order to heal it, you are going to need to reopen the wound, let out the infection and remove the splinter.

This is not a perfect analogy, because you will never be able to remove the experience from your past, however what you can do is change the way you view the experience, learn to accept that it happened and that it is a part of you. It should not have any bearing on the way you choose to live your life from this point forward.

Reopen the wound

Reopening the wound is the acknowledgement that the pain exists, and the exploration of the event and the pain that it caused. You have already done this. You recognized the pain, discovered where it came from and explored the past experience that hurt you.

Let out the pain

The pain started with the feelings that you had. You did not or could not express them at the time. It has grown to include any feelings that you have developed in the time since the incident(s).

One way to begin to heal is to talk to someone about the pain you feel from your past experiences. If you are in a safe environment speaking with a counsellor you trust, you can voice your anger about what happened to you. Unleashing anger is not an excuse to become aggressive. Never direct your anger towards a person. Direct it toward inanimate objects. You can hit pillows, punch your mattress, or go to the gym and punch a punching bag, write about it. Find a healthy and safe way to express it.

Venting anger does not necessarily make the anger go away. Venting can relieve the symptoms. Processing personal experiences, seeing concrete change, and genuine forgiveness helps the anger to go away. To further rid yourself of the pain, you can let the person or people who hurt you know how they hurt you in a verbal and non-violent way,

One way that you can do this is to write a letter, or write several letters. Write each letter in the first person to give a voice to what happened to you in the past.

Address your letter to a specific person. You may need to write to more than one person. It could be a parent, an ex-partner, or any other person from your past.

While some people choose to give the letter to the addressee, you may choose to use the letter as a tool to help yourself. You may want to avoid a confrontation if you are worried the other person will not be able to give you what you need. Sometimes, the person you are writing it to may no longer be available.

Ask yourself, "Is it important to me that the other person knows how he or she affected me or is it enough that I give myself a voice?" There is no right or wrong way.

Write whatever you like. Some general ideas to think about include:

- What did you need from the person that you didn't get?
- What did they do to you?

- How did their behaviour affect you?
- Add anything that you feel you want to express to the person. A story, or maybe a situation?
- Speak from your heart. Speak from your feelings.
- If this is comfortable for you, let the other person know that you no longer need him/her.
  You can also include that you have yourself now and you will take care of yourself.

Your letter might read something like this:

Date …
Dear Mom, Dad, (or insert a name):
I want to tell you what it was like living with you …
I remember when …
This is what you did to me …
This is how you treated me …
This is what you would say to me …
This is how I felt about what you did to me …
This is how I felt about how you treated me …
This is how I felt about what you would say to me …
This is what I needed from you …
This is how it affected my life …
Signed,
Your Name
© 2016 Francesca Tomas All Rights Reserved

This is the core part of the healing, to let the hurt be heard.

If you choose to confront the person, you can use the letter you have written as a guide to help you with what you need to say.

You may need to write several letters before you are satisfied.

If you were traumatized as a child or raised in a dysfunctional home, you may be stuck with feeling that you lack power and hope. Now that you are an adult, understand that you now have power and hope. YOU get to decide your future. Your choices come from the adult you, not the child in you.

You are going to stand up and say, "That was not okay with me." The goal of writing this letter or these letters is to express the feelings, getting them out of you and onto paper. Let them know what it was like for you, what you experienced during the trauma, and what you needed from them.

You may think something like, "Whoa! If I said that to my mom, there is no way. She would just freak!" Remember this letter is about your feelings and you are entitled to them. It is not about worrying about how it will affect the other person.

If you feel that confrontation could hurt the other person, you may choose to not give the letter to him/her. It may not be a letter to pass on to the recipient. You do not need to give it to anyone. You just need the courage to write it down. Sometimes, it is better not to confront the person because you may not get what you want from them. If they were not able to give you what you needed then, they are unlikely to be able to give it to you now.

One of my clients did not care anymore about what her mother thought. She expressed her anger to her mother. She was not expecting her mother to change or to give her anything. She just needed to stand up for herself. After she did this, she felt relieved and empowered with her mother-daughter relationship. That was a big turning point for her and her mother.

If you decide to confront your father, your mother, your lover, or anyone else who hurt you, it is best not to expect that they will hear you and acknowledge their part in your experience. This may not happen. Be prepared for this. It can potentially hurt you if you have high expectations. If you want to confront the ones who hurt you, it is your choice. The letter writing exercise is very effective by itself. The act of putting the words down on paper unburdens you. Once you are unburdened, it becomes easier to accept that you are unable to change the past. Accept it and move forward in a more positive direction.

Here are some examples of letters my clients wrote to various people in their lives:-

Steve had a very difficult childhood. His mother drank heavily, and did not pay any attention to him. He did not receive the care that he felt he needed as he was growing up. He wrote this letter to express the anger that he felt about the way his childhood was.

Hey Mom,

You need to know how angry I have been with you through the years. In fact, angry doesn't even begin to grasp how I've felt. At times it's more like infuriated. You make me so mad sometimes I want to rip my eyes out. You pretend to be two different people that changes on a whim. You pretend to be loving, caring, apologetic and blissful, then suddenly hurtful, vengeful, cold and aggravated the next. You have been like this my entire life.

It's hard to believe anything good you ever said to me because just as fast as something diplomatic is said it is later a sham to the merciless insults that follow. I have always felt like I have never truly had a mother. No support and a deep overwhelming feeling of alienation isn't exactly a great way to grow up, is it?

I sincerely feel you are a horrible person who has nothing to live for and must spread misery like a plague. Still you feel it's necessary to try to bring me down with the ship. You are like the Titanic stuck in a time loop unable to sink. You tell me to do something with my life but what have you done? You have no friends, a job you hate and constantly complain about and no passion for anything other than your next drink. I would have rather been raised by sheep. Congratulations.

Your legacy of pain cannot last forever. Your days of transferring your own feelings of inadequacy, powerlessness, fear, hurt and anger are coming to an end. I think I have got something out of all this after all.

How NOT to live life.

Sincerely,

Steve (A better person than you)

....

Another client grew up with a father who ignored him, and barely even talked to him. He essentially had no relationship with his father. This client never felt loved or accepted by his father, who only ever made demands of him, on the rare occasions that the father spoke to the client.

Dear Dad,

We have never been close or had any sort of positive relationship. Even as a kid I felt it best to avoid your presence. I was always aware of your presence and always leery of you. I never felt comfortable around you or wanted to talk to you. Every time you called my name I knew it was either because you wanted me to do something or to lecture me. We never shared any real good memories.

I just grew up thinking it was normal for kids to not talk to their parents. When I saw other kids and the way they were closer and more open with their parents I realized that this wasn't normal. Over the years I have built up tremendous animosity and anger towards you and the entire family. So much so that I am now ready to love on my own and cut you out of my life.

My relationship with you has had several consequences for me.

1) I feel I am becoming or have become a very negative or cynical individual such as yourself.

2) I never feel good enough and feel like I have something to prove and feel I have to keep my guard up.

3) I have a hard time making any new friends and feel like I'm better off alone.

4) Your high expectations of me have caused me to feel ashamed of every job I have done even when I know I shouldn't be.

In short, I feel I got nothing positive from being your son. You were a good provider but a lousy father. I sincerely hope I don't become like you. Most of my memories of you are poor ones. Even the time we did spend together was full of activities that no child would want to participate in, like yard work, construction, etc. I feel you were more like a boss than a parent.

Sincerely,
Your Son

....

This client struggled with addiction for many years beginning when he was a young teenager. He wrote this letter to the stepfather who had abused him physically and emotionally as a child, and continues to be emotionally abusive, despite the client now being a young adult.

Dear Don,

I am writing you this letter for the sole purpose to let you know how your anger, depression and negative behaviours have truly affected me. Your disregard for my feelings frustrates me and leaves me feeling worthless, empty, lonely and pushed around. Since I was a young innocent boy, your verbal abuse and put-downs have further lowered my self-esteem, making my confidence shrink.

I try my very best to treat you with respect, kindness and love, but time after time you hurt me by belittling me and making me feel like a piece of shit who was never good enough or up to par with your nephews and nieces. I'm truly sorry for all the pain I've caused you in my self-destructive years of addiction. Sometimes I feel you can't forgive me. There's nothing more I want than to make you and mom proud. It's something I work towards.

I feel the way you act towards me is very cruel, I'm sure you love me. The way you show your love I feel is very unusual. Your mean nature has long lasting effects on my mind and negatively changes my mood and stirs up my emotions.

I appreciate a lot of the things you do. You give me advice and input on various situations and lifestyle scenarios. You cook the family fabulous dinners and support the family by going to work and maintaining a successful job. You're also there for my mom. Even though you're often mad and angry, I truly believe you mean well.

I hope one day our relationship is better and less bitter and toxic. I'm going to do my part to better myself because it takes two to tangle.

Sincerely,

Dave

....

This is another piece of work from the client mentioned above. He also wanted to express some things to his father, however he felt that he could not write a letter. In this instance, I asked him questions, and he answered them. This is a rough transcript of that dialogue:

F: Can you tell me what your dad did to you?

D: You gave me drugs, when I was just a young teenager. You neglected me. You disappointed me.

F: How did you feel about what he did to you at the time?

D: I felt abandoned and lost. I was confused, let down and hurt.

F: How has this affected you?

D: It made me a different person. I would have better self-esteem, if you hadn't done what you did. It made me an angry person. It made me not care about myself, and it made me not love myself. It made me self-medicate and it made me feel lost.

F: What did you need from your father?

D: I needed love; a good father-son relationship. I needed a father, not a friend. I want you to take some responsibility for what you did. I needed guidance and help.

F: What would you say to your dad?

D: You are a lousy dad. I love you because you're my dad. It was not okay to hurt me. I am angry with you. You are a shitty role model. You are an alcoholic. You should never have been a father.

....

You can also write a letter to a persistent issue that you've been having, such as an addiction, anxiety, or an eating disorder. Here is an example of a letter like that.

This letter was also written by the client who wrote the letter to his stepfather, and was featured in the transcript of a dialogue we had, that you just read.

Dear my addiction,

I really hate you. You have made me a junkie and ruined my life due to your extreme lifestyles. Because of you I've repeatedly lied, stolen and manipulated my friends and family to get money for drugs.

I've indulged in multiple types of crimes including drug trafficking, robbery, and shoplifting to get my hands on pills and powders. People don't trust me. I'm often called things like lost cause, addict, junkie, scumbag, and drain on society because of my actions.

When I truly give in to you, I will do almost anything to get drugs. Our relationship is toxic, unhealthy, sick, dismal, and dark.

When I don't have drugs, I feel sore, hurt, depressed, sick, down and unmotivated and too unenergetic to do anything. You made me lazy and sluggish, feeling often like a broken, crippled old man in a wheelchair.

My dependence on you again and again has me lost in a vicious cycle of the struggle. I feel helpless against your powers.

You have not only sent me into a downward spiral but you have affected my family by showing them what hell on earth really is and displaying it in front of their very faces. I hope you leave my body and mind and let me live life like it is supposed to be lived.

Sincerely,

Dave

....

It doesn't necessarily have to be a letter. Here is a poem a client, Archie, wrote about the bullies from his childhood.

BULLY

Although I ignore you, I still live in fear
Although I deplore you, I still shed a tear
There's nowhere to run, and nothing I can say
There's nowhere to go, to take away the pain

And I don't find this funny at all
Because I can't climb over this wall

Over my dead body I will hate you
Over my dead body I will forsake you
Over my dead body I will forgive you
Over my dead body I will forget you

I'm so afraid of what I've become
I pray every day for my kingdom to come
You'll never know what I conceal
The hand of God is cold blue steel

Now you don't find this funny at all
Because you can't climb over this wall

Over your dead body I will hate you
Over your dead body I will forsake you
Over your dead body I will forgive you
Over your dead body I will forget you

Here are two more poems, both written by the same client, who had a very difficult childhood. Her mother used to wake her up in the middle of the night to beat her, among other things. These poems are not addressing anyone in particular, however they are a way she used to express her feelings about the turmoil she experienced in her early life.

CLOSED DOORS
Kim Robin

She hides behind the doors
Of yesterday's sorrows...
She tries so hard to open
Maybe one slowly, then two
For possible tomorrows...

She says please step inside
But will only allow you so far
If you try to get to know her
She will flee...................
                          And shut the door.

Her pain and hurt are deep within
All the doors that protect her...
Hard and solid, tough and strong
Like a blockade which allows no

One to pass.

Underneath is a child so small
Who steps forward trusting and
Loving.....................
But is betrayed..................
And each door
Closes behind her.
The innocence she once held
In her eyes...........
Are clouded with deception

Through a peep hole... She tries
to see the world again
So she opens each door and steps through
Her footsteps feel scared and afraid
But she pushes each door.... Wider and
Wider..................................
She trusts herself now and knows she
Will never......................
Hide behind closed doors.
....

TOUGH TEARS
Kim Robin

Tough tears are the ones you cannot see
But inside their drenching me
I walk around and pretend they're not there
I won't let you see them I won't even dare

For friends to turn to
I always listen
I'm always there
Remember, I always did care

I cry and feel for whatever you're going through
But who was there
Who really even did care
When I needed someone to turn to

The subject was changed without despair
As if it wasn't brought up
Like it wasn't even there.

I'm tough & strong for all to see
But does anybody know the real me
I'm tired & sad
And want to let go

Guess I'm just lonely
And need someone to care
If I turn to you
Would you be there?

I stand alone like I always do
I wish that someone would reach out
But they never do…..
……..

Forgive them when you're ready

Forgiveness does not mean the experience was OK. It means you don't want to carry the pain anymore. You have a deeper understanding now. You see the pain inflicted on you was really the other person's pain that they passed on to you. It wasn't about you! You are in charge of what happens next for you.

Grieving

To fully heal, you may also need to grieve and mourn that child in you who didn't get their needs met, and was hurt or abused. Grief is a mixture of sadness, emptiness, and the feeling that you have lost something. Mourning is how we express our grief. This is a natural and essential part of healing.

To grieve, there are some things that you should do. The most important thing is to acknowledge the pain. It is a part of grief and a necessary step on the path towards acceptance and healing.

It's a good idea to get support from a friend, a loved one, or even a counsellor who can be there for you while you experience all of the emotions that are a part of the grieving process.

It is also important to take care of yourself while this process is occurring. Feeling all of these emotions can take a toll on you, as it requires a lot of energy.

Try to ensure that you eat well, sleep enough, and engage in some physical activity every day. This will give you the extra energy to work through it.

Frequently, the hurt starts in childhood. I suggest that you "the adult" write a letter to you "the child"– your inner child. This is a great way to acknowledge the pain you may feel; to grieve for the child that you were, and the person you might have been.

Write to your Little Self and let him/her know that you are here for them now. Tell the little person inside. "I'm here for you, and nobody knows what you need better than I do."

You can also write a letter to your adult self from your inner child.

When you write the letter from child to adult use your non-dominant hand. If you're right-handed, write the letter with your left hand. This allows you to access the child in you more easily. It will come out like a child writing.

Your Little Self can tell the adult you what it was like to go through the experience. For example, "I was scared, I was horrified, I was hiding under the bed when I heard Dad and Mom fight all the time. When I heard Mom being punched I would hide."

Sometimes you may fear the feelings that will come up when you look at your memories of that time you were hurt and you try to stay away from them. Know that you have lived through the experience, the memories will not kill you. Working through the pain will help you move forward. You have made it through the traumatic incident.

Now you will take yourself through the experience in a different way. The purpose of writing the letter is to finish your past once and for all and to give yourself a voice. You are standing up for your inner child and for yourself as an adult.

As a child, you may have not known how to defend yourself or to walk away from the situation. You may have felt powerless or even hopeless. As the adult, you do have power and you do have hope. You can walk away. As an adult, it is important to take care of your inner child that lives inside of you, it is up to you to give him/her the emotional support and care that perhaps you did not get when you were small.

If you were abused as a child, you may be stuck there. Finish your past and let go of the negative effects of the experience. You can then move forward into your future, feeling empowered and in control of your life. The letter enables you to become an adult.

Let out what you felt – like worthless, helpless, isolated, or abandoned. Voice all the things you have never given voice to. Face them and allow yourself to experience the feelings.

Depression, anxiety, and addiction may come from denying the expression of these emotions and the release that comes with it.

Here is an example of a letter that a client of mine wrote to a younger version of herself. Her family moved around a lot, and she started to use drugs and be promiscuous at a young age. She eventually was sent to a youth correctional center, due to breaking the law as a teenager. It was there that she met her husband, and they both turned their lives around. Because of her past, she has fears that she will over parent, or that she will do something that will cause her children to be taken from her. She regularly fears that something will go wrong and she will lose all of the things she has worked hard to gain since she made the decision to change for the better.

> Dear Me,
>
> I am not sure when or how it all started but I remember how every step felt. I am not sure why it always comes back as bad. I am not sure why you always focus on the bad stuff but it's ok. I can tell you that it does all work out good. You must have always surrounded yourself with negative energy. Maybe that's why so much bad stuff always seemed to happen.
>
> Good stuff must have happened. You just don't remember it. I know that when you were given choices at such a young age you had too much control and lost all sense of being a kid. That really sucked. Then you felt so alone that any type of attention was wanted so bad, but it wasn't the right type. THAT'S NOT YOUR FAULT. You did choose to be left alone. You made the best decision you could at that time and it's OK.
>
> When you finally were on your own, another one who gave you the wrong type of attention came along.

All you ever wanted was for him to love you. I think in his own way he did, he was never taught to show it. But he still managed to make you feel like garbage when he had sex with someone else in front of you, because you were menstruating, THAT'S NOT YOUR FAULT. It's OK. You did leave and that was for the best. All the ones after that were just filling an empty hole but you did not create that hole. Other people left that hole in you. That's not your fault.

So don't blame yourself. You dealt with it as best you could and that's ok. When that didn't pan out you found something else to make you feel good over the next few years and men. You dabbled and people liked you because you always had drugs. You were the party girl but everyone always wanted to be around you, that felt good. When that fell apart and you got kicked off the track nobody came to your side. Once again, totally abandoned. THAT'S NOT YOUR FAULT.

So on to the next person to make you feel needed and wanted but they just used you as well and when it was done yelled at you and told you to go away. So in order to show them that you were capable of being good enough you decided to be a drug dealer. Successful or not they were never going to love you. All the pain and suffering you endured during that time was all looking to help people so they would love you but they never did. THAT'S NOT YOUR FAULT.

Then came James your one love. Even he hurt and rejected you at first. You must have seemed so desperate and you were. Twenty some years of looking for someone to love you and tell you you're a good person. He is wonderful but it still needs to come from you. James' love will never be enough. You have to be OK with yourself, love yourself. You made it through all those years alone chasing and looking for something that you had all along. Self-reliance.

No one survived your life but you. Guess what, you did and great job. You have a wonderful family, home and job. No one gave that to you, you earned it and keep earning it every day.

Don't worry about the things that went wrong, they are in the past. You don't want to miss today because of yesterday. Today you have a beautiful 5-year-old princess of a daughter and a 3-year-old perfect son. No, you can't screw them up because you love them and will never reject or neglect them. Yes, you will make mistakes as a mom but you will always love and tell them every day how special they are. You can't teach them to not make your mistakes or go through what you went through because they will not be raised how you were. They will be raised to know how wonderful they are and to love themselves because they are so loved by you.

Spend quality time every day with your kids and always tell them that they are loved and no matter what they do that will never ever change. As long as you do that they will never go through what you did, so don't worry so much.

Love, Amanda

....

Here is another example of a letter a client wrote to his younger self. He experienced a lot of neglect, and felt that there was always something wrong with him. To this day, in his late twenties, he is still working to overcome the feeling that there is something wrong with him.

Dear Young Steve,

Sitting here it's hard to believe that time has gone so fast. The past just feels unreal and as if it were another lifetime but everything happens for a reason. I remember feeling scared and alone back then. I know it all too well. It felt like you against the world with a permanent sign that said "Kick me" on the back of you. You just wanted to be like everyone else. Having fun, enjoying youth with your friends but it always seemed to be interrupted. What did you do to deserve this you often asked yourself? Nothing. It truly wasn't your fault. You simply existed. You always imagined life differently but it was never what you expected. You felt that things would one day get better but that day never came. You tried to be strong but that only seemed to make things worse in the end.

One day you just lost hope for the future. Nothing you did mattered anymore and you became hopelessly addicted to gaming. You will spend years losing yourself in a dream world of your imagination until you don't know who you are anymore. You will end up making some of the best friends that you ever had and possibly ever will have and for that you are and will be grateful. You felt what little there was left of you was gone. That sense of not belonging anywhere will haunt you for years to come and you will even be afraid to go to school.

Eventually you will get older. Everyone does. You will wake up and wonder where the last 10 years went. Like you just woke up from a nightmare. A real nightmare. You will expect things from yourself and so will others around you. But now facing any part of life is too overwhelming. You feel as though you are walking in a minefield and every move you make leads to tremendous pain, except there is no release from it. Sadness, fear and that feeling of losing control persist like you are slowly losing your mind and have lived inside your head for far too long. Similar to how a schizophrenic patient might feel when a doctor tells them their delusions weren't real. No one can live life vicariously through a computer.

Whether or not I would go back in time and change things is debatable because then I would be changing what it means to be you and you and I both know deep down we don't want that. As you will come to realize how complex life is you will understand that changing yourself will not be an easy task. But if you knew what I know now you would know it can be done with perseverance. Learn to take the good with the bad because there is no one or the other. Life is a battle but it is also beautiful, learn to enjoy it.

Love,
Steve

....

Transforming the way you see the experience

You will never be able to change the fact that your past experiences happened. What you can do, however, is change the way you think about them. You've read some accounts now about how others have done that.

By letting out the pain, the feelings about the incident(s) that you have kept bottled-up, you can see the experience more logically. When you look at it from a less emotionally charged point of view, you can see that while the experience was horrible, you made it through.

You can start to understand that whatever happened to you was not your fault. You did not choose to experience those things, they were thrust upon you. When you realize that your negative experiences say more about the person who placed you in the position you were in when you experienced them, the one who caused the pain, than they do about you, you have taken the first step to remove the splinter. When you can move forward and truly believe that you are not to blame, you have removed the splinter and transformed the way you view the situation and yourself.

Conclusion

Negative experiences from your past will continue to cause you pain until you deal with them. There are several steps to take.

First, acknowledge the experience. Go back and examine it and your feelings about it.

Second, release the feelings and the pain that you are holding from the experience(s) by talking to a counsellor and/or using the letter writing exercises.

Third, transform the way you view the experience and yourself. Recognize that you are not to blame. Do not allow the negative experiences to define you.

Next, we will look at some important findings from my years of experience, in relation to strong negative emotions, and the defence mechanisms people employ when they experience them. People employ both unhealthy and healthy defence mechanisms. In the next chapter you will read about both kinds, and some ways to transform your use of unhealthy defence mechanisms into healthier ones.

Chapter 7
Healthy Defenses

"Only when we are no longer afraid do we begin to live."
– Dorothy Thompson

Introduction

Now that you have started to deal with the pain your past experiences have caused and have transformed the way that you think about them, it is time to examine your present. The hurts that you felt affected the way that you deal with things that happen in your life now. They influenced the way you react to negative emotions.

Now you will look at some of the reactions you may have had and learn about some of the defense mechanisms that we use to deal with negative emotions. Then you will learn how to transform your own unhealthy defense mechanisms to healthy ones.

When you feel a strong emotion like fear or loneliness, what do you do?

One way that you may cope with strong feelings is to shut them down.

As soon as you feel uncomfortable, you may also feel uncertain about how to deal with the emotions or how to "get out" of them. Your temptation to escape will continue until you understand that both fear and loneliness are shame-based emotions. They each have a powerful effect on your emotional wiring.

This "escape" pattern may have started in childhood, especially if your parents had difficulty navigating their own emotional minefields. They did not have the skills to teach you how to navigate yours.

When you are a child, you are unable to say, "Mom and Dad, I know you're dysfunctional, so I'm moving down the street. The Smiths seem like they're much better adjusted." You can't really say that so you just stay where you are. You cope in whatever way you can. Often, the easiest way to cope is to shut down your feelings. We learn this technique very early in our lives. What happens when a child experiences a traumatic event and no one there offers support? That child will find a way to cope, usually by shutting down his/her feelings or by acting them out in some negative behaviour.

Many people cope by ignoring or pushing away difficult feelings. As a result, they may develop an addiction to a substance or behaviour to help them cope with the difficult feelings that they are trying to avoid. They may just put up with bad feelings or negative behaviour and think "This is just the way I am" or "This is just the way that life is." They may fall into one of the patterns linked to unhappiness. These patterns may include the need to stay busy, to move from place to place, to go from relationship to relationship, to become a perfection-ist, or to become a controlling person.

If this sounds like you, and you want to change your life, sooner or later you will have to deal with the underlying issues. Often, people reach the point of needing to resolve these behaviours because of a personal crisis.

Fear, Loneliness, and Shame

The roots of the word *shame* are thought to derive from an older word meaning 'to cover.' 'Covering oneself' literally or figuratively is a natural expression of shame.

Many of our undesirable behaviours are rooted in shame. These include: addiction, the need to control, perfectionism, poor self-esteem, overachievement, power seeking, anger, jealousy, self-hatred, aggression, social anxiety, and withdrawal from friends and family.

Have you ever experienced any of these? When were you shamed? Shame is usually developed when you are the most vulnerable. For example, you may have asked for help in a math class. Instead of receiving help, the person you asked to help you ridiculed you instead and said that you were stupid.

Often, parents are not perfect either. When your mom or dad did not give you enough time and attention, you may have felt "I'm not important enough. I'm not good enough. I'm not worth my mom and dad's time." This could be shaming.

Were you ever hit, beaten, or verbally abused when you made a mistake as a child? Abuse in any form is shaming. Sexual abuse is very shaming. For the most part what you can't talk about or think about is what shamed you as a child.

When we do not learn healthy coping skills for stress or for a traumatic event, we often develop defense mechanisms. Most of these defense mechanisms are unconscious. We don't even realize that we use them. Some of us use denial to keep us from the truth and help us to defend our idea of who we are.

Some Defense Mechanisms

What follows are some of the unhealthy defense mechanisms many of us use:

Denial

Denial is refusing to accept reality or fact. We use denial to avoid the truth about what may have happened or to avoid feelings that are painful. Denial keeps us safe. When we refuse to see reality, it keeps us from having to confront it. For instance, a person who smokes marijuana daily will deny that he or she has an addiction. If you question this, the person may say "Everybody does it" or "It's not harmful" or "It's legal." This denial does not change the fact that this person is addicted and is unable to get through a day without this "fix."

Projection

Projection occurs when your thoughts and feelings are seen as unacceptable to express or you feel uneasy about having them. For example, a wife accuses her husband of having an affair. Actually, the wife is the one having an affair and is diverting her feelings of shame or guilt towards her husband.

Dissociation

Dissociation occurs when you are not connecting to your memory, your thoughts, and your own sense of identity. For example, a woman tells her counsellor, "I think my uncle may have exposed himself to me as a child, but maybe I just dreamed it." This shows that the woman may not be connected to her memory of the event, and may be unconsciously protecting herself from the painful memory.

Dissociation has been clinically linked to painful past experiences. Childhood abuse, especially chronic abuse that started at an early age, has been related to high levels of dissociative symptoms. Memories of abuse can trigger amnesia. Adult women have been found to have increased levels of dissociation if they were sexually abused by a much older person before the age of fifteen.

Dissociation is also linked with a history of childhood physical and sexual abuse and increases with the increased severity of the abuse. A 2012 review article supports the hypothesis that current or recent trauma may affect the way someone thinks about the distant past, changing their perceived experience of the past, and resulting in dissociative states.

Reaction Formation

Reaction formation occurs when you change unwanted or dangerous thoughts, feelings, or impulses into their opposites. For example, a woman who is very angry with her boss and would like to quit her job may instead be very kind and generous toward her boss and express a desire to keep working there forever. She is unable to express how angry and unhappy she is with her job. Instead, she becomes overly kind to publicly demonstrate her happiness and her lack of anger.

Rationalization

Rationalization occurs when you offer a different explanation for your perceptions or behaviours when you see that reality is changing. For example, a woman who has been dating a man she really likes, and thinks the world of, is suddenly dumped by the man for no reason. She changes the way she views the situation in her mind by telling herself, "I suspected he was a loser all along."

Defense mechanisms are often a learned behaviour. As an adult you can work with a professional counsellor or other healthcare professional to learn how to use healthy defense mechanisms that could help you more than the unhealthy ones you may currently employ.

Some healthy defenses are:

Sublimation

Sublimation occurs when you change unacceptable thoughts and emotions to ones that are more acceptable. For example, a man who is having thoughts that he knows he should not act upon may intentionally refocus on going for a walk or going to the gym.

Assertiveness

Assertive behaviour includes the ability to stand up for your rights without violating the rights of others. Assertiveness falls in between passive and aggressive and is the most desired communication skill. It is also the most helpful defense mechanism for most people to learn.

Now it is time to figure out which of these mechanisms you use. That is the first step in transforming them. When you are able to recognize the patterns of your defenses and the situations that lead you to use them, you can examine why you use them.

Many times, the reasons for your defenses are from the wounds that you have learned ways to heal in the previous chapters. Often you will find that you use unhealthy defense mechanisms less frequently, as you heal the wounds from your past. This allows you to consciously move towards using the healthy defense mechanisms.

Becoming aware of the mechanisms that you use most frequently is a great first step. When you catch yourself using or about to use an unhealthy defense mechanism, attempt to use a healthy one instead. This is not something that will happen immediately, it is a process. *Transformation doesn't happen overnight.* The more you examine your responses and work on substituting healthy defense mechanisms for unhealthy ones, the easier it will become.

Conclusion

Many of the negative behaviours people exhibit are rooted in shame, fear, or loneliness. We all use defense mechanisms to help us cope with these unpleasant emotions. Some of these mechanisms are healthier than others.

When you start to heal the wounds of your past, you may find that the unhealthy defense mechanisms you use occur less frequently. You can also consciously work on changing the mechanisms you use by being aware of the types that you gravitate towards and the situations that usually prompt their use. Then make an effort to use the healthier defense mechanisms when those situations arise.

Be patient with yourself. Changing behaviours takes time and effort. It may not happen as quickly as you would like. You will likely see progress soon enough.

Next, we will look at how to take action to change your life now that you have learned how to be self-reliant. You have worked to transform the way you think about the past, and the way you react to situations in the present.

Chapter 8
Take Action

"We must be willing to let go of the life we've planned,
to have the life that is waiting for us."
--Joseph Campbell

Introduction

Now let's focus on moving forward as you open yourself up to new life experiences. It is time to begin to live in the moment and enjoy yourself. You have come a long way and can now trust your ability to be self-reliant. Stop waiting and start doing!

Take action and move forward in your life

Taking any action in your life will get you moving in a different direction. You do not even have to know exactly where you're going. It doesn't matter if you have figured out a clear direction. Do something different. When you make a move, you will realize you are not stuck any more.

As you know from my personal story, there were times when I simply walked into something because there was nothing better to do. Those "accidents" turned my life around for the better.

Yes, it is good to have goals. It is also good to open yourself to the many possibilities around you. When you take chances, you can make changes in your life.

Pursue your goals with a sense of openness and adventure. Leave yourself open to opportunities and possibilities that might come your way. Sometimes life takes you in a direction and you just have to follow and not get too attached to a specific outcome.

Follow your instincts. They will tell you when you absolutely must do something that has come up. For instance, you may take a job knowing you won't do it for life, but it could have potential. Maybe a stepping-stone that can help take you to where you really want to go. Perhaps you will have more opportunities there.

Try to remain open to opportunity and change. If you are too inflexible, you may miss opportunities that will help you reach your goals. Make different choices by opening up your world.

Many of us live in a very small world we have created. The whole rest of the world is out there to explore. Decide to get out and try something completely different. Look for venues where you can find like-minded people. Commit to try some new activities and connect with other people who have similar interests.

To get a different result, you must try something different. If you do this, you may have to go into new territory and this could make you feel a little apprehensive. Stick with it. The rewards can be amazing.

It is okay to feel uncomfortable. Nothing is going to change unless you change it, period!

That is what taking action is about. You need to recognize what you need and completely take charge of your own life. It takes strength and courage. That is the only way you are going to change things in your life and find freedom and happiness.

Do not just keep doing what you have been doing. ***Stop!***

Do something that takes you in the direction you choose. When making a decision, here are some questions to ask yourself:

Will this choice lead me in the direction I want to go in?

Is this choice going to take me away from what I want and need in my life?

Is this choice going to keep me stuck repeating the same pattern that is causing me the problems I am trying to prevent?

If you do this, your life will take a different direction.

When you want to make changes in your life, it is important to have a plan. The following is a step-by-step guide to the creation of such a plan.

The 'Take Action Plan' to Change a Behaviour

Creating a '*Take Action Plan*' is a useful way to understand the steps you need to take to achieve a goal, such as changing a specific behaviour. It can be adapted to work for most goals.

- Clearly state the goal you want to achieve.
  o Example: I want to start a career

- Why is it important to you?
  o Example: I want to feel fulfilled and have a stable income

- Why does it matter to you?

- o Example: I want to be independent and know that I can take care of myself and be successful.
- • In point form, specifically state what you have to do differently.
  - o Example: I need to make a decision as to what kind of career I want.

I need to get training in my chosen field, so I need to research places that offer training

I need to stop finding excuses to put it off because I am afraid I might fail

I need to apply to a training program for my chosen field

I need to work hard at my training and keep myself on track, by avoiding things I know may cause difficulties

If there is more, keep writing until it is clear to you what you need to do.

Let life take its course

Accept where you are right now, but know the direction you want to go in. Look and see if there are some changes you can make. Creating change comes from trusting yourself, taking chances or trusting the universe or a greater power that life will take you where you need to go.

Be present in each moment. Be aware, and open to possibilities that may come your way. Countless people have said that this has worked for them. I see people find jobs, make different choices, and have things go in the right direction for them.

Live in the moment

When you live in the moment, you will find it enriches your experience. If you over think how you could have done things differently in the past or if you become anxious about the future, you will find that being present lessens this kind of worrying.

It is not a bad thing to examine our past and learn from our mistakes, or to plan for our futures. When you spend the majority of your time dwelling on what might have been or have negative thoughts about what might be, these thoughts are not going to lead to happiness or satisfaction.

For example, a lot of women go on a date with thoughts like, "I hope this relationship is The One," or "I think this is the one I'm going to marry," or "I think this one will work out." It's not advisable to begin dating someone with that expectation. You put too much pressure on yourself and may set yourself up for a big disappointment.

You may want to approach dating as an opportunity to get to know the other person, to enjoy their company and the moments you share. Stay in the present.

Wherever it goes, it goes, and you might be pleasantly surprised. Know that whatever the outcome is you will be OK!

This approach will really tamp down your anxiety about dating and about being with people you don't know well.

Trust Yourself

Only when you admire your own beauty and appreciate your true self will you start to resonate with all that you are doing. You will be confident that you really are a good person. Feeling good about who you are comes from you, not from someone else. You can rely on your gut instincts. They will guide you in the right direction. Know that you can trust yourself to do what you need to do for yourself. You are the expert in your life.

Conclusion

In this chapter, you have learned to take action to change behaviours and change your life. Remember to take life as it comes. Live in the moment and trust yourself.

Chapter 9
Live Up to Your Expectations

"Holding on is believing that there's only a past;
Letting go is knowing there is a future."
– Daphne Rose Kingma

Introduction

In this chapter, I share some of the most important findings from my years of therapeutic practice. I have worked with many unique clients. Each client comes to me with a different situation. However, common themes frequently surface. There are certain aspects of our lives that many people struggle with, that we are constantly striving to improve. In this chapter, we will look at these areas and the positive results that can result after working through the S.T.A.R. system.

Live Up to Your Own Expectations

You must be willing to disappoint your parents. Many of us grow up trying to please our parents. Now, you may be trying to gain the respect of someone else in a position of authority, like a teacher or a coach. It is only natural to try to conform to the standards your parents set. You can end up living your life from where you were raised, what you were told, and what you saw growing up.

When you try to live up to someone else's expectations, you have a tough task. Even when you think you have met or exceeded those expectations, the other person may still not give you the credit you feel you deserve. Even if you get the approval, you continue to feel unfulfilled. This may lead you on a constant search for approval.

Remember to live **your** life. If you don't, you will continue to feel defeated as you try to live up to your parents' or someone else's idea of who you should be or what you should do or not do.

Maturity occurs when you decide that you need to live your own life, even if you know others do not agree. You remain a child as long as you need constant approval from people other than yourself. What matters is how you feel about the choices you are making for yourself. If someone does not agree with the choice you made, that's okay.

Parenting

The best gift you can give your children is to become a healthy complete person yourself. This is critical. Children look to you to be confidant, to understand, to know how to express love and to model how to be a man or a woman. It is not enough to just say, "Now this is how things should be." You must *live* it too!

If your life is out of control, how can you expect your children to be in control? Yes, parenting is a big responsibility, but it is also a very rewarding experience. Children can be a big incentive to become a better person. Good parenting comes from fully expressing yourself in a positive, loving, and respectful way. Not putting expectations of your unfulfilled life onto your children.

If you love and respect yourself, your children will learn to love and respect themselves. They do this in two ways. They observe the way that you show yourself love and respect, and how they receive love and respect from you.

When we do not work on our own pain and deal with it for ourselves, we can unconsciously pass that pain on to our children. It is important to be consistent in the messages that we send to our children with both our words and our actions. If we tell them to do things one way, and then proceed to do them another way ourselves, this can cause confusion and create problems for the child.

Inner Wellness

Many of us believe that satisfaction and approval will come from achieving great success, having more stuff, and being financially successful. The truth is that many people who achieve this financial status are still not happy.

At the end of the day, they still feel empty and struggle in relationships. Emotional wellness does not come from things and money. Having a comfortable life can relieve financial stress. Less stress may contribute to a better life. But it isn't everything. Inner wellness comes from knowing that you matter, that you are a worthy person just being you. And you really like who you are.

What are some of the signs of inner wellness? Are your relationships about love, kindness, giving of yourself, giving and receiving emotional support from the people that matter to you? Feeling a sense of inner peace versus conflict. You trust yourself to do what is best for your own well-being and for the people you love. You do not beat yourself up if you make a mistake, instead you learn from your choices. This is emotional wellness.

Are you happy with the choices you have made? Do you have a purpose in your life and are you fulfilling it? Your purpose can be anything you choose from being a great parent to becoming a great financial advisor to being a great artist. You decide what your purpose is.

For the most part, society tells us that being educated and wealthy makes us important and more desirable. It is wise not to make financial and educational success your only identity. If you do, you are likely to attract those who have also made it their identity. It is important to make emotional wellness a bigger part of your success. If you think money and material things are all that you need, think again.

I have met and counselled many clients who are educated and financially successful and yet do not know who they are and struggle with themselves and in relationships. Putting all your energy into what you do versus who you are can become problematic later in life.

Intimacy

Intimacy comes from Latin intimus and means "closeness."
Intimacy is often a difficult topic. It implies letting someone else get close to us to see all of our secrets and hidden places. An intimate relationship means that we are willing to let go of our defenses and be seen by another for who we are. This includes seeing all of our vulnerabilities and weaknesses - which can be terrifying.

If you are hiding something from your past, this can create a barrier to an open and intimate relationship. If you are unable to accept this hidden past yourself, you may think that it is nearly impossible that someone else will be able to accept it. This is because most people can sense when people close to them are uncomfortable about certain aspects of their lives.

You experience intimacy when you have a close, familiar, and usually affectionate or loving personal relationship with another person. You may share dreams, thoughts, feelings, and sadness. You may give emotional support to each other.

Be willing to set your own goals based on your true desires. Be willing to walk the road less traveled to please *you.* If this means disappointing your parents, or someone you care about, understand this could be a necessary step on your journey to emotional self-reliance.

We all need to be compassionate and try to understand our parents and our partners. That does not mean you should give up your dreams, your life, or yourself to please another person. Being true to who you are and living the life you want is important for you to feel good about who you are. When you realize that you can't be the person you want to be because you are trying so hard to be what everyone else expects you to be, you may begin to feel off balance, unhappy, hopeless, and helpless.

We all work the same way

All of us work the same way. We have been taught to believe that men and women are different and want different things. My experience working with both men and women is that we are more alike than different.

We collectively believe that men have more affairs because that is "just what men do." Men are hard as steel - men don't need to hear positive words, praise, and acknowledgment. Men don't hurt like women when a relationship fails. They can handle rejection better than women. Men's feelings don't get hurt like women's feelings.

From my experience counseling both men and women, I have found that men hurt just as much as women do. Men want a loving relationship just as much as women do.

For many men, appearing strong and able to handle a broken heart or a disappointment is what men feel they are **supposed** to do. They may believe that their job is to take care of a woman's feelings.

What we believe about men may be wrong, just as it is wrong for us to believe that a women's job is to do housework, or to take care of the man of the house. These are traditions that no longer serve us today.

We all need to feel that we are important to our partners. We want to feel that we matter, that we are appreciated, supported, accepted, and understood. We want to be validated as good enough exactly as we are. These are basic human emotional and social needs, for men and for women.

Both men and women come to see me in my practice to discuss self-esteem issues. The more you understand yourself and accept yourself as you are, and make the changes you need to make that will get you to where you want to be, the fewer anxiety or mood issues you will have. Often low self-esteem is linked to issues such as anxiety or depression. By increasing your self-esteem and accepting who you are, you are taking steps toward overcoming your anxiety and/or depression problems.

When you recognize the factors that may have been affecting your ability to take action, and you have worked through them, you have undergone a transformation. You can now move forward.

Relationships

Do you struggle in your relationship because your emotional needs are not being met? Are your expectations of your partner reasonable? Your relationship can not give you everything. There are qualities we should look for in our relationships that are a must. Mutual respect should be the foundation. If you are fighting and not happy in your relationship, you may be trying to get something that you were denied in childhood out of your current love relationship? Unconditional love, understanding, value, trust, validation.

Are you repeating a family pattern? Look at your relationship; is it similar to your mom and dad's relationship? What you grew up with becomes your normal today. If you were looking for attention, unconditional love, and understanding from mom and dad, chances are you could be looking for your partner to fill those emotional needs for you. The irony of this is that for the most part we will end up with a partner who also is unable to give us what we need emotionally. We repeat patterns in relationships in order to try to get it right through our partners. If you are able to get from your partner what you did not get from mom and dad, then you may feel unconsciously, "I am worthy." Or you may continue to fight it out because this is what you know and/or you yourself don't feel worthy of love.

This is why loving and respecting yourself in every cell of your body is so important. If you love and respect yourself, then you will not allow anyone who does not show you love and respect into your life. *Like attracts like.* Relationships can teach you about yourself. What you allow or do not allow in your life is in line with how you feel about yourself.

Enjoy the results of all your hard work.

The outcome of this difficult soul-searching work can be a fantastic game changer for your life. You will be able to live the life you want to on your terms. You will no longer be constrained by the patterns that you developed in reaction to your past trauma. You have dealt with the issues that have been causing you problems and can move forward, with a new healthier outlook.

Yes, other issues may reveal themselves. However, now that you have learned healthy ways to deal with your issues, and you know there is positive growth ahead, you can do it again and again.

In 'My Story', my walk across a bridge became an important and transformational event. Seek and find those experiences that will enrich your life. Remember that even if you lose your way for a time, you will bounce back stronger.

Conclusion

I hope you feel encouraged and motivated. I have covered some tough topics. You are not alone. The issues that you face are being faced by people everywhere. All of us are human and we suffer in similar ways. Although the pain can be similar, each story is different. Take comfort in this. With the right approach, you can overcome obstacles and reach toward a better and happier life!

Chapter 10
Success Stories

It is important for me to emphasize that *many* people struggle with a difficult past. Many decide to make peace with these struggles and experiences and move towards a more positive and rewarding future. Below, I have included the story of a few of my clients with their permission. They have both used the steps in the STAR system and the letter writing technique. These are success stories that I hope will motivate you to heal and grow personally.

Shaun's Story

I was born in 1982. I was raised by my mother and step-dad. Although born in Vancouver, BC, I was raised all over the lower mainland. My parents were alcoholics and addicts, so these issues were in my life from very early on. I have witnessed some horrific things that I now know.

I have seen my step-father overdose twice. I can still remember him at the bottom of the back stairs doing the flop and turning blue. I was probably 10 or 11 years old and in fifth grade. My brother and I learned to pick the lock to the downstairs room where they kept the presents and found pounds of weed and a lot of cocaine with needles.

I remember confronting my mom. She said she would quit. A few months later, I stole some weed to sell to my friends. I stayed at my friends' houses, pretty much living with them, when I was still in sixth grade. I started hard drugs and heavy drinking by eighth grade.

I ended up in juvie and was court ordered to live at my mom's. I can't remember what I did. During that time, my mom and step-dad split up. My mom and I started dealing together, her at the bar 16 hours a day, me at school and at home. That's when it really spiraled out of control with new "friends" and new criminal escapades.

My true friends and my older brother came to my house and punched me out. He made me pack some clothes and drove me straight to Calgary, where I turned 18. When we arrived, I walked into the house and it was a grow show. I watched people get stomped for collections and saw a few shootings. My house was raided and I moved back eight months later.

When I came back, I moved in with my grandmother and started closet smoking crack with my uncle. I started grade twelve at the age of 19 and my grandmother died. I then dropped out of school, boozed it up and got high for the next five years.

During that time, I started as a simple cracker, selling all of my valuables. I moved into a crack shack and became a doorman. I started selling drugs on the street to feed my own addiction. A successful, non-smoking dealer "invested" in me and showed me better methods. Soon I had my own houses that I ran.

I met my wife in one of these houses and I remember being so successful. I had tons of dope and money. I was staying safe and hiding it because eventually you fall asleep and someone steals it all. I have stayed awake for days always making money, but being an addict you can count on always being around other addicts.

An easy pay day was all anyone wanted. I woke up to having nothing more than once, even missing my shoes or my hats. Sleeping with whatever you had stuffed in your underwear or socks, just to wake up to nothing. For me it was a business and an addiction, but you work for 3 or more days, then fall asleep and have to start all over. I'd had enough, but my wife kept going, and so did I.

We stopped working the houses, just tried supporting our own habits. But without an income from dealing, you do whatever you have to do. Within six months I was arrested a number of times for possession, trafficking, and robberies. I was accused of driving for bank robberies and armed robberies. I was questioned about murders and other people I had started to associate with.

While I was in jail/pre-trial, I proposed to my wife. When I was released a few weeks later, I received a Father's Day card. I never wanted to be the parent that I grew up with. For me it was a pretty easy decision, no more dope. That was a whole new struggle. Getting into and actually going to a recovery house was the hardest thing. The fact that my girlfriend/fiancé was going with me was great motivation, but the stigma and stats around couples getting clean together was overwhelming.

I started working and drinking more often to help stay off drugs. We got married while in recovery and moved to a house that we shared with my younger brother. I then started drinking even more and began to smoke weed. I got drunk and relapsed.

My daughter was born in February of 2008, and I had had enough with court issues, so I fast tracked all my cases and started **pleading**. I was charged with a robbery, possession, and a trafficking charge. I received a three-year Conditional Sentence Order, which is like house arrest. I had a curfew, but was allowed to work.

I BLEW IT. I got drunk, relapsed, and went to jail. I went to jail for my remaining time of eight months. While there, I went to Alcoholics Anonymous, Narcotics Anonymous, and Anger Management. When I was released I was given conditions, one of which was to see a counsellor. We found Francesca. My wife found her for me, and I still see her today. She was and is an amazingly huge part of my sobriety. She has helped me to better understand why I always backslide into drugs, and has taught me better coping skills.

I am now 31 years old. I have been married for seven very short years. I have a six-year-old daughter, and a four-year-old son. I live in a nice house, own two vehicles and have two dogs.

My biggest advice is this: *Fix your past for yourself, and the future can only get better.*

....

Archie's Story

I'm an addict, but I don't do drugs, drink alcohol excessively, gamble, hoard, steal, or overeat. I'm a recovering pornography addict.

As a boy, I would sneak into my parent's room to look at my dad's *Playboy* or *Penthouse* magazines. As a young man, everyone I knew looked at porn, shared porn, and made jokes about porn, at work, at home, at parties. And when the Internet arrived, it was everywhere and anywhere, 24/7. It still is.

I've always been compulsive about certain things, like completing a project, learning a new skill, or getting through all the levels of a video game. My compulsive behaviour is another sobering realization of how addicted I was to pornography. It was like collecting stamps. I spent hours upon lost hours downloading and organizing only to delete everything later out of shame and guilt. Then I would repeat the cycle over again. The time I wasted I will never get back – time I could have better spent with my family.

I don't know exactly when my addiction started, but it was likely around the time my life started to go sideways. Before 9/11, life was good. I left my office job and started my own business. My wife and I were making good money and we were planning to buy a house and start a family. Soon after, contracts were cancelled, business dried up and our first child was born. I couldn't find a job and my wife learned she couldn't have any more kids.

Broke and nowhere else to go, we moved back in with my parents. It was the most humiliating, depressing and stressful period of my life. As I slid further into depression, I hid in video games and porn. Like all men are taught, I did my best to pretend I was strong, act like nothing was wrong, or blatantly lie about what I was really doing. I didn't realize it at the time, but I was heading deeper and deeper into a very dark place and getting very little sleep.

One of my earliest memories is being afraid of my grandmother. I still have a memory of her leaning over my crib yelling at me. Something terrible happened to me as an infant in my grandmother's care because I was always petrified of her. I don't remember what it was, but it was severe enough that my parents left our country and moved to Canada.

I can imagine the fear and excitement my parents felt being in a new country with small children. Although it was not easy, I'm sure they felt relief being far away from a toxic environment. Unfortunately for me, things were about get worse.

From being beaten by teachers and bullied by kids at school, to being molested by my parent's new friends, I lived through horrible circumstances growing up in a new country without aunts, uncles, cousins, grandparents, and not many friends. Was it really that much better so far away from my scary grandmother?

When I started school, the real torment began. There were no ESL programs and "the strap" was still in place. I was different, spoke a different language, and took longer to answer questions and write tests. I was an easy target.

My parents, God bless them, did the best they could. Trying to fit in, they taught me never to fight back, to turn the other cheek and take the high road. The bullies, they assured me, would eventually leave me alone.

Unfortunately, the opposite was true. Walking away meant I was a coward. I came home many times bloodied and bruised. The few times I did fight back, I ended up being swarmed the next day, often pinned down while the swarm took their turns. Eventually, I was the one who had to learn to take it, because everyone who is different gets beaten up. That's the way it is.

The bullying got so bad, that by the time I started high school, I wanted to kill every bully in my school. Had my parents kept guns in the house, I would either be dead or serving life a sentence. I didn't care about the consequences of murdering my tormentors. I just wanted the pain to go away.

While the images are blurry and sketchy, the feelings of living in constant fear, loneliness, and humiliation are all still very real, even today. The helplessness and hopelessness from being in a school system that provided little support for immigrant families left a deep and nasty scar.

After high school, I thought all my troubles would be over because the bullies would be out of my life. But the imprint of being constantly beaten and ridiculed for being different destroyed whatever self-esteem I had left. Looking back, I can now see I merely cast those skeletons aside, hoping to never see them again. I never dealt with my shame properly. How could I? My role models were as much ashamed as I was.

Little by little, as my life continued to unravel, those skeletons reared their ugly heads. Shame, fear, and lack of self-worth drove me to self-deprecating behaviour. Sometimes I didn't care. I wanted to die. But then I'd see my family happy and playing together and I would cry. What was I doing? More importantly, why?

One day I woke up scared and felt that what I was doing was not normal. Like all addictions, my addiction to porn was seriously undermining my health and my relationships at home and at work. It also never occurred to me that the women I was looking at were getting younger, not older. And even though most of the images I was looking at were like Playboy magazine "erotica", the nude models were now under 18. That scared me because I knew where that was heading. What was I thinking? What was wrong with me?

The best thing I ever did was pick up the phone and call for help, because I was heading down a dangerous rabbit hole that I was not able to climb out of by myself. I needed help.

For the past four years, counselling has helped me work through painful childhood memories and how shame has shaped my low self-esteem and negative thinking. I see how my unhealthy habits were cries for help and that what happened to me as a child was not my fault. I am worthy, I belong, and

I matter, like all of us do. More importantly, nude images of women under 18, sexually explicit or not, is just wrong. It's not normal.

I love my parents dearly. They did what they thought best by taking their family to what they thought was a safer place. But during that transition, they bestowed their own shame upon me, hoping to protect me. Instead, like all enablers do, their good intentions enabled the torture and ultimately the addiction.

Counseling and therapy has shown how I was heading down the same path of transferring shame upon my own child as my parents did with me. This has been the most enlightening lesson for me personally. I can see how obsessed I was about protecting my family from bullies and that I was making my shameful experience theirs too. I was completely blind to it, thinking I was doing them a favour, when in fact I was actually doing it more for myself and to justify my behaviour.

All my life I have felt uncomfortable asking for and accepting help. Reaching out and asking for help is not a sign of weakness. It's a sign of strength and maturity. The help I get makes me feel better about who I really am, one day at a time. I deserve better. Everyone deserves better.

For the first time in my life, I'm beginning to like who I see in the mirror.

About the Author

Francesca Tomas has been assisting her clients with their transformations for the past 10 years as a Registered Professional Counsellor, a Registered Therapeutic Counsellor, a Life Skills Instructor, Empowerment Coach and a Group and Workshop Facilitator. She holds certificates in Trauma, (PTSD) Disordered Eating, Motivating Change, and Mindfulness Counselling.

This spring Francesca will be launching
her powerful new Signature Program called
"90 days to Bold, Beautiful, and Strong!"

www.followyourownstarcounselling.com
counsellingsurreybc@gmail.com
604-314-8063